AF824489

Praise for William Reiley Butler and this book

Closing relevant remarks by Joyce Kulhawik at a woman-owned business seminar: *"Ladies, get a second or third opinion! Second opinions and informed medical advice is crucial to the information-gathering and decision-making process all patients should engage in as they take charge of their own health."*

~Joyce Kulhawik/ Emmy Award-winning Broadcast Journalist and 3-time cancer survivor

"Even if you are comfortable and fully trust the doctor diagnosing you, get a second and possibly third opinion, as it may save you from pain and suffering in the future. It did me."

~Kim O'Brien, a patient in the book, who by acquiring three opinions were saved from years of disability.

NAVIGATE
THE
MEDICAL MAZE

Indispensable Resources and a Roadmap to Explore the Critical Importance of Second Opinions from Hospitals, Surgeons, Rehabilitation Facilities and Caregivers

BY
WILLIAM REILEY BUTLER

Copyright © 2021 by Life's Realities Press and © 2021 William Reiley Butler

ALL RIGHTS RESERVED. This book contains material protected under International and Federal Laws and Treaties. Any unauthorized reprint or use of this material is prohibited. No portion of this book may be used, reproduced, stored in a retrieval system, or transmitted in any form or by any means — electronic, mechanical, photocopy, recording, scanning, or other — without express written permission from the authors or publisher, except for a brief quotation in critical reviews or articles. It is illegal to copy this book, post it to a website, or distribute it by any other means without permission from the authors and publisher.

Published by

Life's Realities Press
Westborough, Massachusetts
Publisher William Reiley Butler's information: https://william-butler.com/

Copyright Use and Public Information

Unless otherwise noted, images have been used according to public information laws.

ISBN: **978-0-578-95207-9** Paperback

Limits of Liability and Disclaimer of Warranty

The author and publisher shall not be liable for the reader's misuse of this material. This book is for strictly informational and educational purposes.

Disclaimer

The views expressed are those of the author and do not reflect the official policy or position of the publisher or Life's Realities Press. This publication is designed to provide accurate and authoritative information regarding the subject matter covered. It is sold with the understanding that the publisher is not engaged in rendering legal, accounting, clinical or other professional advice. If legal advice or other expert assistance is required, the services of a competent professional should be sought. The opinions expressed by the authors in this book are not endorsed by Life's Realities Press, and are the sole responsibility of the author rendering the opinion.

DEDICATION

I would like to dedicate the content of this book to...

My brother Lanny Butler who called me once a week during my years of operations and physical rehabilitation. His advocacy and support were life-saving.

Val Kearns, Don Hanssen, Mike Rizzo, and Pat B. for their visits to the rehabilitation facilities and my house. They arranged food when I could not walk, provided good conversation, drove me to medical appointments, and gave me small gifts which raised my spirit.

Kim O'Brien who experienced the need for second and third opinions to save her quality of life. Kim, instinctively, sought additional opinions that were later used in this book.

Carol Isvak who became my partner after all I went through. Her support, suggestions, and acceptance of my crippled body is true. I never thought it would ever happen.

My brother John G. Butler Jr. whose story is used in the book to promote acute care second opinion and what to look for. I miss him.

ACKNOWLEDGEMENTS

Friends, Family, and Patients

Billy Butler – advocate. He raised money through GoFundMe, from friends and family so the book could be published.

Hannah Rubin – advocate. She designed and posted my current website, william-butler.com

Carol Isvak – home care advocate and contributor

Pat Sr. – contributor who worked at the YMCA

Rich D. – acute care contributor

Catherine Johnson – rehab. facility friend, advocate, and bingo partner; may God rest her soul

Jonathan Rizzo Foundation – assists those in need in memory of Jonathan Rizzo and I was one of many the foundation has helped

Stacy Drake – advocate and contributor

Barbara Butler – contributor

Jennifer Grippa – contributor

Gary Lowe – advocate. He made sure that my car was ready and waiting when I could drive again

Kim O'Brien – a multiple opinion contributor and advocate

Henry Agri – friend, advocate, and contributor

Don and Ann Hanssen – contributors and advocates

Medical Professionals - The doctors, surgeons, registered nurses, Certified Nursing Assistants (CNAs), and others:

Dr. William H. – orthopedic surgeon

Dr. Phil A. – orthopedic surgeon

Dr. Julie W. – infectious disease

Dr. Perez – infectious disease

Dr. Cliff, Chris, Bani, Lisa, and the staff at UMass Memorial Medical Group – Westborough, Massachusetts

Dr. Edward Hoffer – contributor

Dawn Swanson – contributor

Valerie Kearns – advocate and contributor

David O'Toole - Contributor and advocate. David assisted in my discovery of the Medicare.gov/care-compare.

Lorna Doane – A Boston registered nurse working with patients, doctors, surgeons, and staff in various hospitals.

And all the medical professionals, hospital/rehab/home care patients, and roommates who need to stay anonymous. Thank you.

TABLE OF CONTENTS

Chapter One: Hope — Fight — Live 1

Chapter Two: Inpatient Rehabilitation Facility (IRF) or Skilled Nursing Facility (SNF)...............95

Chapter Three: Pain and Communication 149

Biography of William Reiley Butler.. 187

CHAPTER ONE

HOPE – FIGHT – LIVE

Due to my first infection in 2011, I had a near-death from a spinal operation. After three weeks of corrective surgery from the botched operating room process, I opened my eyes. The ICU nurse said, "He is going to live. Pull life support!"

After the 2015 and 2017 hip implants, I contracted bacterial infections in both hips. It was undeniable that I would die if the infections were not eliminated. Anyone who has battled cancer, sepsis, and other deadly infections and disease will place great fear upon receiving a positive test result. Waiting for a phone call from your primary or specialist doctor on test results is surreal.

> *At the YMCA, a friend of mine told me that cancer patients refer to this feeling as "Brain Stop." Thoughts of the future are replaced by emptiness. All your plans or projects are suddenly put on hold or stop altogether. It is a waiting game.*

There must be *hope,* trust, and a belief that the situation will have a positive outcome. The people I have spoken to found that hope is worth *the fight.*

To have another chance, you must trust that the medical professionals will get you through. If you cannot count on the professionals and your own will, you could not only lose because of the final diagnosis but because you convinced yourself that all hope is lost.

Optimism must be a part of the cure. Once you are informed that you will *live*, plans for your future will start again. Pain, suffering, and the process you endured will remain in the past. You did it; you lived!

Fighting includes due diligence. Yes, you must trust the professionals, but only if you have consulted and interviewed their "equals."

Surrounding ourselves with support from friends, family, religious organizations, and disease support groups can weaken fear and strengthen hope. Any positive approach will be beneficial.

If a friend, family member, or acquaintance speaks of adverse outcomes, should you distance yourself from them? If you want a negative reality, let the medical professionals have that discussion with you. Few things are worse than listening to an acquaintance talk about how bad their experience was having a baby while a woman who is pregnant is present. The same holds true when a person has an infection or cancer.

The importance of an advocate

The patient advocate can be defined in several ways. ... They obtain medical records, ask questions, keep notes, help patients with difficult medical decisions, and review and negotiate medical bills. Often the patient advocate is a close friend or family member who is not paid for their service. Oct 5, 2016 Healthcareitnews.com

I was fortunate to be introduced to Dr. Edward P. Hoffer, who graduated Magna Cum Laude from Harvard Medical School and worked at Mass General Hospital in Boston. Dr. Hoofer is a cardiology specialist and general medicine expert and has carried out research studies on cardiovascular systems.

Dr. Hoffer suggests in his book, *Prescription for Bankruptcy – A doctor's perspective on America's failing healthcare system and how to fix it*: "[I]f you end up in the hospital, try to have a friend or family member by your side as much of the day as possible. If permitted, have them get you up and frequently walk during the day."

An advocate who is positive, objective, and helpful will assist in taking charge of your medical decisions. They could save your life.

Types of advocates: An advocate can be a friend, family member, nurse, doctor, or paid service.

Support from an advocate: An advocate could provide the most-essential questions, advice, and answers through their notes and feedback. For example, the advocate can be the stenographer. While you learn from the doctor and then respond with questions, you will not be sidetracked by writing notes yourself. All of your attention will be directed towards the doctor's behavior and the content of the consultation.

The objective of an advocate asking questions is to assist you in making a thorough comparison of hospitals and surgeons. You are the one who must decide, unless there is an unforeseen incident that needs acute care immediately. An advocate's support will help you prepare physically and mentally, gain confidence, and increase hope.

I was extremely fortunate to have two advocates, Pat B. and Don Hanssen, during my last four hip operations. During a consultation with a surgeon at one of the finest orthopedic hospitals in the country, I asked the question, "While having a spacer in the hips, what is my mobility? Will I be able to drive a car?" The doctor demonstrated that a leg should only be able to bend 5 to 10 degrees. He mentioned that just getting into a car would bring difficulty, let alone driving the vehicle.

Not only did this terrify the hell out of me, but it also delayed an operation to eliminate a deadly bacteria. Pat and I decided to head to the second surgical team (and a different HMO) on my list.

The second medical team disagreed with the first. The head of orthopedic surgery said, "With rehabilitation and physical therapy, mobility and flexibility will be restored upon having the spacer and using tools. A physical therapist will teach you how to enter and exit a car and work with you so your range of motion will be adequate."

Using crutches, I drove my car safely, walked with 50% weight-bearing, and sat comfortably. My range of motion was 45 degrees or more.

I decided on the hospital that saved my life due to their presentation and the surgeon's control. When I met with a lead orthopedic surgeon at Newton, he was front and center while his team circled to the right and left. The team was asking questions and conversing about my history and medication. After a comment by the lead surgeon at the end of the consultation, I decided after a comment, "Okay, team, I want ideas on how to approach this, on my desk by the end of the week!"

At that point, my confidence soared. He meant business, had all the authority, control, and most importantly, the responsibility for failure.

Pat B. wrote down what was said and the behavior of each of the three surgeons I consulted. The two other hospitals and surgical interviewees were skeptical about the outcome of a double revision. Even their tone of voice and behavior showed a lack of confidence. Pat's notes captured many items I might have missed. Pat's notes were pivotal in my choice to have the best surgeon and team.

Asking questions before the operation and during recovery is a must and is a right. Without an advocate, I might have missed an answer or behavior that would complicate my decision.

Pat Sr. is an acquaintance I met at the YMCA in Westborough, Massachusetts. He is a Shihan in martial arts and a Marine. Pat told me during an interview, "It was my mother-in-law and my wife who insisted that I elect to have an amputation below my knee. They were my advocates, and they stayed by my side throughout the process."

In Pat Sr.'s case, his mother-law and wife were the advocates pushing for an operation, and Pat agreed with them. His advocates were family members, and they helped save his life from progressive infection. If you can acquire an advocate, listen to them. If you do not have an advocate, seek one out. Once Pat Sr. listened to his advocates' hope for him, they raised his confidence to a level that let him make a medical decision that changed his life forever. As a result, he is happy, functional, and has a good quality of life.

Seek out the Healthcare Advocate: The responsibility of a healthcare advocate "is to help patients navigate the stressful financial aspects of the healthcare system. This includes educating patients on reimbursement, billing, and financing options. Healthcare Advocates also have extensive knowledge of insurance plans, their coverage options, and limitation." online.utica.edu

If you are going to be hospitalized, seek out the healthcare advocate where you will be treated. Hospitals and rehab facilities often have healthcare or patient advocates who will help with finances, insurance, post-hospital care arrangements, and more. Their advice could save you and your family a significant amount of money and stress.

If the hospital or rehab facility does not advocate for patients, ask a trusted family member, friend, or medical provider who already knows you to help you in that role.

Be your advocate: The definition of self-advocacy is "speaking up for yourself, making your own choices about your life, learning how to get information so that you can understand things that are interesting to you, finding out who will support you in your journey, and reaching out to others when you need help and friendship." (www.medicalhomeportal.org)

Lea, a registered nurse from Boston, commented, "If there is no support locally or you are alone on the path of surgery, be your own advocate. Ask questions and make doctors accountable for the good *and* the bad!"

Later in the book, you will read about Larry T., a patient who confronted his nurse because she brought him the wrong pills. It took him an hour to convince the head nurse and the floor nurse that he was correct. Finally, Larry said, "Bill, you have to be your own advocate."

I had no advocate from 2011 to 2018 until Pat B., Don H., and Mike R. in 2019 and 2020.

Even if you have an advocate, sometimes you still must speak up for yourself. I had such an experience during the last days of my stay at CareAll. My assigned nurse stopped my last four antibiotic Vancomycin IVs and was working on discharging me that day. I knew there must have been a misunderstanding between the infectious disease doctor (and CareAll), who told me that I needed four more intravenous treatments. I wheeled my wheelchair to the main nursing station. I insisted that the orders were for more antibiotics. The logistics manager took it upon herself to call my infectious disease doctor, Dr. June Wind, who confirmed that I needed four more IVs.

In my mind, those final IVs may have been the amount required to kill the infection. By challenging the nursing staff, I was correctly administered the necessary medication, which I knew the doctor ordered. My feeling is that the last application of Vancomycin most likely saved my life.

After reading a medical journal, I was impressed by their list of seven ways to be an advocate.

7 Ways to Advocate for Your Own Health Care

1. Do not be afraid to ask questions! Ask about the benefits, side effects, and disadvantages of a recommended procedure.
2. Understand how your health insurance works.
3. Do your research!
4. Maintain your records.
5. Get a second opinion.
6. Review your medical bills for errors.
7. Know your rights at work.

(May 4, 2018. www.arthrosurface.com) and (http://www.ndalc.org/)

Multiple opinions save lives.

In 2011, I worked out at the local YMCA, bent over, and showed signs of pain or discomfort.

A man approached me and asked why I was in so much pain. I responded, "My spine has lost the cartilage between disks, which is irritating the nerves all the way down the legs. So, I'm having a spine operation next month." He asked, "Where is the operation?" I responded, "A hospital in Worcester, west of Boston." He answered, "Do not go. Get a second opinion somewhere. Talk to New England Hospital in Boston." I was curious, so I asked, "Are you a doctor?" "Yes, I am," he said. "Where?" I asked. "At the hospital where you have scheduled your operation. You will never come out the same!"

I did not take that doctor's advice. I contracted two infections during the operation and/or during post-operation. I became a cripple. In the hospital records, the infections were described as "Staphylococcus bacteremia complicated by nosocomial pneumonia and acute pleural necrosis." I learned later, through research in medical articles, that you can only get the infection bacteria I contracted at a hospital.

Lives nearly lost by lack of good opinions: You may say that this could never happen to you, yet this book will contain the experiences of at least four disabled patients who listened to friends, family, or their primary doctors but never took the time for a second opinion. Three are disabled, and one died. The questions are how to narrow your choices down to three options, and what techniques or resources should you use?

In a paper entitled "Incidence of Staphylococcus aureus infection after Elective Surgeries in the U.S. Hospitals," by Jill Dreyfus of Premier Applied Sciences, published by Oxford

University, tied infections to surgery and/or post-operation care: "risk of post-surgical infections can be related to operative procedure/technique, duration of the surgery, perioperative control measures, post-operative care, as well as patient demographics and health status."

Her conclusion about healthcare-associated infections (HAI) was, "Our results highlight the need to improve existing surveillance methods and find new strategies such as vaccination after surgeries."

In my case, the right hip deteriorated, and the pain was unrelenting. The hospital I chose was recommended by a lifelong friend who had success with their orthopedic department. The surgeon was professional, but I did not get a surgeon's second opinion. The final result was two infections, one in each hip. My friend Don was just attempting to help me. It was not his fault; it was mine. It was my responsibility to receive a second opinion.

The surgeon who operated called me and gave me the bad news. "Bill, you will need a double revision, and we cannot perform one at our hospital. You need to investigate other surgeons and hospitals."

It became apparent that the infections had to be eliminated, or I would die. This time, I visited three hospitals and three surgeons. All were under different HMOs. It was the second hospital out of the three that I choose to help me. I honestly believe if I had not chosen one of the other two, I would have died of sepsis. The surgical team and the infectious disease doctor saved my life. Or did I save my own life by diversifying my options?

We will follow Kim O'Brien's journey through her decision to have multiple opinions after recognizing a spinal problem. As I mentioned before, I declined the idea of a second opinion before my spine operation and suffered dire consequences. Kim, a schoolteacher in Richmond, Virginia, gathered three specialists from her primary and then had to navigate the paths to either lifelong disability or a successful outcome and good quality of life.

Ms. O'Brien wrote, "The symptoms were: Dizzy spells, tingling/numbness in arms, legs, and face. Very mild pain in the neck area, muscle tightness, and occasional mild nerve pain.

"I started feeling dizzy and numb in my arms, legs, and face six months before surgery (November of 2014). I went to my primary care doctor, and she prescribed steroids and sent me to a neurologist. The neurologist ordered an MRI. She was suspicious that my neck might be playing a part in the symptoms and looked at the brain. The MRI showed severe degeneration in cervical discs C 5–6 and C 6–7. She sent me home with the names of a couple of orthopedic surgeons and neurosurgeons that the doctor had worked with in the past. I trusted her opinion since I taught her children in elementary school for years."

I must be clear that you may not have three surgeons to examine you. If you live in a rural area, access to multiple hospitals, surgical specialists, and HMOs may be limited. If you can drive or fly to another town or city and get that second opinion, your life could depend on it. "Selecting surgeons, hospitals, rehab facilities, and home care" will now provide criteria for making decisions. You are not limited to these ideas.

On page 118 of *Prescription for Bankruptcy, America's failing health care system and how we can fix it,* Doctor Hoffer talks about information-gathering before choosing the hospitals and surgeons to visit. "When you want information about disease or treatment, always start at the most trusted site, run by the National Institutes of Health: https://www.nih.gov/health-information. If you do not find what you need there, go to a site maintained by a large, trusted hospital system such as Mayo Clinic, Cleveland Clinic, or Massachusetts General Hospital."

In Doctor Hoffer's opinion, "If it is a serious diagnosis and major interventions are proposed, do not hesitate to ask for a second opinion. Good doctors should not be offended by this. Second opinions often change your care. Remember: It is the doctor's job to help you. It is not your job to make the doctor feel better by offering blind trust."

You must request your records: It is imperative to request your records after every consultation with your primary doctor, specialist, practitioner, surgeon, and testing department. Records should include notes the professional has put into their system, notes and pictures from blood tests, X-rays, MRIs, CT scans, preparation documents, operation notes, post-operation records, and DRG codes. The healthcare records created by the medical professional system are your property. You have the right to the records and supporting documentation due to HIPAA, a federal law that sets a national standard to protect medical records and other personal health information.

In my case, a significant complication developed during the 2011 operation on my spine. It was not until 2016 that I asked for all my records. Don Hanssen, my advocate, and I read about the seriousness of the infections and why they occurred. Since I had become crippled, I needed to organize the records and highlight the justification for Social Security Disability Insurance (SSDI) coverage. Thanks to doing that research and getting those records, I received SSDI benefits on my first request.

Why your records are essential:

- To understand the diagnosis and the reasons why
- The records can be given to other medical professionals for your care
- Detail the process, what happened, and who was involved
- Will be used for qualifying for SSDI should there be complications
- To request a change or amendment to your medical or billing record if it's incorrect
- For documentation should a legal dispute arise

The reason why the Diagnosis-Related Group (DRG) codes are important is that "DRGs allow the healthcare provider to provide more information on the severity of your illness within the group and allowing CMS (Centers for Medicare and Medicaid Services for health coverages) to adjust costs based on different stages in the progression of an illness or complications or comorbidities (CCs). Minimal or maximum coverage based on the DRG codes written in the system by the surgeon and staff." Carevoyance.com or verywellhealth.com

You may need them or never even read them, but your records are your property, and your right.

A hospital resident who took the time to listen to the patient: Don Hanssen, my advocate, and his wife, Ann, provided a true story about his father-in-law. "Henry was a healthy 87-year-old senior living in Fort Myers, Florida, who ate well, didn't smoke or drink, worked out three days a week, and always went for a walk or bike ride after dinner. In November of 2015, he started complaining of vertigo problems and went to see his family doctor. He was given an antibiotic for an ear infection and told to drink plenty of fluids. After his vertigo did not go away, Henry returned to his doctor, who said vertigo is common in seniors and suggested he have his hearing aids checked."

When Henry's family visited after not seeing him for six months, they were concerned about his walking. He walked amazingly fast with his head down; when asked, Henry said he always felt like he would fall over if he did not move quickly. They urged him to see a specialist and get an MRI. Instead, his doctor sent him to a balance clinic specializing in helping people with similar issues. The clinic said an MRI was not necessary (after all, he was 87), and many seniors have vertigo and prescribed a series of head and eye exercises along with a regime of walking three times per day.

After several months and no improvement, his family was appalled that he still had not had an MRI. But being of the old school, he assured them his doctors must know best.

One night on his evening walk, Henry fell and cut his hand. Fortunately, his neighbor was a nurse who convinced him that the wound required stitches, so his wife drove him to the local hospital. The resident who came to clean and stitch the wound started talking with Henry about what happened. During the next 45 minutes, he listened to a seemingly healthy and cognizant 87-year-old describe his last nine months of dizziness. "Did you ever have an MRI?" "No," Henry replied, "the doctors never ordered one." "Well, you are going to have one now," he replied, and Henry was wheeled away.

Later, the resident returned with a neurologist. The MRI showed a brain tumor the size of a golf ball, and Henry needed immediate surgery. He was moved to a different hospital, where a neurological surgeon determined that waiting was not an option even at 87; they operated the following morning. Thankfully, the biopsy showed that the tumor was not malignant. However, the type of tumor was extremely fast-growing, doubling in size every month. In recovery, his surgeon said that he would have died within 30 days, given the aggressive growth, without the surgery and a resident who listened to the patient.

Henry recovered fully and is doing quite well at 92.

COVID-19 is an exception: When the United States shut down in March of 2020 because of the COVID-19 pandemic, the Centers for Disease Control (CDC), hospitals, and emergency organizations quickly put together appropriate admission techniques. It took time to create a process that the population could follow. In the meantime, hospitals were flooded with those who needed immediate attention and people who were fearful of virus's symptoms. The rehabilitation facilities were accepting potential COVID-19 residents and/or had patients who were already infected. Hospitals were at capacity and locked down the rehabilitation facilities and nursing homes. However, it took months to realize that residents were already infected, passing the virus to others and dying at a high rate.

COVID-19 is the exception when you do *not* have time to investigate opinions and options for hospitalization and rehabilitation. As time has gone by, medical professionals and patients learned how to prevent the virus by cleaning the body, using masks, protecting the eyes, staying home, and identifying the symptoms that require immediate hospitalization.

New home point-of-care test kits have been approved for use. The test kits could be the exception to the rule for planning what hospital you would like to care for you. When symptoms or what you think are symptoms develop, you can test yourself. The data will be sent from the test kit to the medical professionals. Knowing this device is available and distributed, it would be prudent to choose the facility before testing positive and hospitalize if the symptoms reach a critical stage, so you have the time for research before you must take immediate action.

"Now, more Americans who may have COVID-19 will be able to take immediate action, based on their results, to protect themselves and those around them," said Jeff Shuren, M.D., J.D., director of the Food and Drug Administration (FDA) Center for Devices and Radiological Health.

We will review the symptoms, stay-home decisions, and preparation for optional hospitals and rehabilitation facilities before admission. Then, you can use the same methods described below in decision-making for COVID-19.

Selecting a Hospital

Here are techniques that individuals in the book and I used for evaluating hospitals. However, I am sure that additional processes can be used for deciding on the three hospitals that you and your advocate can investigate. You should use them if they seem appropriate.

Ways to search for a hospital include the following.

Family, friends, and primary physician: A standard method for selecting a hospital is to listen to people you know and trust. Based on the praise of a hospital by those individuals who had a good experience, you may narrow down the three hospitals to visit. Your primary doctor's recommendation is a way of adding to the three options. Often, a primary or specialist doctor will put in a good word for a hospital and surgeon in the same HMO.

It is highly recommended that the three hospitals on your list do not belong to the same HMO. The HMOs rely on their databases and processes to assist in the care of a patient. By diversifying your investigation and consulting with specialists at different HMOs or hospital systems, there is a greater chance of an accurate diagnosis, leading to more hospital choices. When your primary doctor suggests a specialist, that specialist typically works within their hospital system. Your primary physician may be motivated because they can be involved in working with the specialist, visiting the hospital, and controlling all reports.

Should you only take your primary's recommendation, you are at risk. It may comfort you that you have your primary physician and the same hospital system. Still, without investigating alternatives, you have lost the chance of missing a more capable specialist who may provide better care and save your life.

Medicare.gov/hospital/compare: Hospital Compare has information about the quality of care at more than 4,000 Medicare-certified hospitals, including more than 130 Veterans Administration (VA) medical centers and more than 50 military hospitals, across the country. You should use Hospital

Compare to find hospitals and compare the quality of their care.

Medicare comparison is in partnership with the Center of Medicare and Medicaid Service's (CMS), which reinforces the focus of *Selecting Surgeons, Hospitals, Rehab Facilities, and Home Care* and its objective of investigating opinions.

The information on Hospital Compare:

- Helps you make decisions about where you get your health care.
- Encourages hospitals to improve the quality of care they provide.

In an emergency, you should go to the nearest hospital. If you can plan, discuss the information you find here with your healthcare provider and be prepared to decide which hospital will best meet your healthcare needs.

Hospital Compare opens new windows in collaboration with organizations representing consumers, hospitals, doctors, employers, accrediting organizations, and other federal agencies." Learn more in the Guide to Choosing a Hospital. Their website explains: "The methodology uses a statistical model known as a *latent variable model*. Seven different latent variable models are used to calculate scores for seven groups of measures.

1. Mortality
2. Safety of Care
3. Readmission

4. Patient Experience
5. Effectiveness of Care
6. Timeliness of Care
7. Efficient Use of Medical Imaging

"The overall hospital quality star rating is calculated using the hospital summary score.

"Only hospitals with at least three measures within groups or categories, including one outcome group (mortality, safety, or readmission), are eligible for an overall hospital quality star rating. Not all hospitals report all measures. Therefore, some hospitals may not be eligible for an overall quality star rating."

An actual comparison of two Massachusetts hospitals: I have compared two hospitals in Massachusetts. I used two ZIP codes: 02120 and 02118. The rating chart is one out of eleven questions of the quality of care to measure.

Depending on your diagnosis, you should thoroughly investigate your hospital options using *Medicare.gov/care-compare*. The tabs are:

- General information
- Survey of patient experiences
- Timely and effective care
- Communication and deaths
- Unplanned hospital visits
- Psychiatric unit services
- Payment and value of care

If Larry, Pat Sr., and I had this data about each of these organizations, our choices would have changed. Taking charge would have saved us from being crippled and avoided periods of torturous pain and suffering.

How do we use the Medicare.gov website: The following should help you drill down into the relevant data you require for hospitals. Note: you can compare more than two facilities at once.

1. *Go to medicare.gov/hospitalcompare.*
2. *Click on "Hospitals."*
3. *Type in the area you would like to investigate (you can choose near the hospital near your advocate and your home. Anywhere you feel the facility you want is located – in this case, zip code 02062/Norwood)*
4. *There are five tabs you can choose from to search/filter criteria you decide to focus on. Distance in miles: Overall rates (star ratings); Other ratings (star rating by categories – Patient survey rating: Timely and effective care; complications and death; unplanned hospital visits; psychiatric unit services; payment and value of care); several beds; more filters.*
5. *The system will provide many facilities to choose from. Click on the first facility you would like to compare. In this case, the 02462/Newton. Then, click the "compare" tab.*
6. *Scroll down till you find the second facility you would like to compare. In this case, zip code: 02062/Norwood. Then, click on the "compare" tab.*
7. *In the upper right-hand corner, click compare.*

8. *The first screen provides relevant data about each facility. Scrolling down, you will find data/information categories to investigate Patient survey rating; timely and effective care; complications and death; unplanned hospital visits; psychiatric unit services; payment and value of care and much more information.*

The following chart contains data from "Patient survey rating and complications and death."

Which hospital would you choose?

Hospitals	Star rating	Death rate from Heart Failure	Death rate for pneumonia patients	C. diff. intestinal infections	Patients who reported the staff always explained medicines before giving them	Patients who report their doctors communicated well	
ZIP code: 02462	★★★★★	8.8	81	.671	67	84	
ZIP code: 02062	★★★	10.3	80	.900	62	79	
National average		11.3	72	1.0 Low better	66	82	

The Joint Commission on Health: The Joint Commission's Website and Quality Check is an internet and voice communication system. You can research the hospitals and doctors deemed capable of performing various operations.

During my training as a volunteer at a Massachusetts rehabilitation facility, the head nurse educated the class about the Joint Commission. She asked about our pasts, so I told her of my near-death experience in 2011 and that they moved me as quickly as possible to a rehabilitation facility after taking me off life support. Her comment to the class was, "I am sure they did; a death would have downgraded the accreditation." I discovered that she was referring to the Joint Commission on Health. The www.jointcommission.org led me to a wealth of information about the measurement of accreditation, specifically, Gold Seal hospitals and their Gold Seal departments.

"The Joint Commission is an independent, not-for-profit organization. The Joint Commission is the nation's oldest and largest standards-setting and accrediting body in health care. To earn and maintain *The Gold Seal of Approval®* from The Joint Commission, an organization undergoes an onsite survey by a Joint Commission survey team at least every three years (Laboratories are surveyed every two years)." (Commission Performance Measurement Data Extract)

Hospitals are required to report three out of five national Quality Improvement Projects: Heart Attack Care, Heart

Failure Care, Pneumonia Care, Pregnancy and Related Conditions, and Surgical Care improvements.

The public can get performance measurements from the internet or by contacting the Commission. Be aware that a hospital can obtain the Gold Seal due to excellent performance on only two or three projects out of the five they provide to the Commission. We can investigate a hospital and learn which of the five projects they earned the Gold Seal through the internet. The question we need to answer is, do those projects match our diagnosed illness?

The field values, explanations, and ratings are (Commission Performance Measurement Data Extract):

- Star = The hospital has met the National Quality Improvement Goal 100% of the time. This is the best, highest-possible achievement.
- Plus = The hospital has performed better than the national average.
- Check = The hospital has performed the same as the national average.
- Minus = The hospital has met the National Quality Improvement Goal less often than the national average.

For example, I met with a South Coast hospital director in Massachusetts during their seminar about orthopedic surgery techniques. He said that his hospital received the "Gold Seal of Approval" and that his department was also in charge of analyzing standard dimensions and their data. The final reports accumulate quality data about the hospital department's data, which the Joint Commission will use for accreditation.

The data are collected and analyzed, and the onsite-visit reports go into the Quality Reporting System to be viewed by the public. A person can determine which of the five Quality Improvement Projects a hospital has been certified for from those reports.

I suggest you go to the Joint Commission on Health's website and click on "Quality Check Website and Quality Reports." You will be able to type your hospital of choice and find the hospital's certifications. (Quality Care website ECO systems) For example, type in Beth Israel Hospital in Boston, Massachusetts. You will see that the hospital is certified in Advanced Comprehensive Stroke Care and Ventricular Assist Device for cardiac circulation, which is used either to partially or entirely replace the function of a failing heart. (Wikipedia)

No matter what method you chose to narrow down hospitals for other opinions, you should review the Commission on Health and similar websites.

Dick Maggio, a successful high-tech executive, had a sudden heart attack. The ambulance and EMTs drove him to Beth Israel Hospital in Boston. Fortunately, Beth Israel has a Gold Seal Cardiac organization employing specialized cardiac surgeons.

Months later, Dick needed another surgery on his heart, and he double-checked Beth Israel Hospital. Dick chose the appropriate hospital for his diagnosis, a decision that was backed up by the Joint Commission website. Dick was then sent to one of the best nearby acute rehabilitation facilities, Braintree Nursing and Rehabilitation Center. On the facility's website, they acknowledged that they were one of six specialties of the rehabilitation center for "Cardiac Care." A perfect fit in both cases. (www.jointcommission.org; www.qualitycheck.org)

Additional websites and patient rights:

www.hospitalsafetygrade.org – The **Hospital Safety Grade** scores hospitals on how safe they keep their patients from errors, injuries, accidents, and infections.

www.abms.org – The American Board of Medical Specialties (ABMS) is an independent, not-for-profit organization founded in 1933 to set professional standards for physician practice and board certification.

Medicare.gov/hospital/compare

https://www.medicare.gov/hospitalcompare/compare.html#cmprTab=2&cmprID=220163%2C220175&cmprDist=9.8%2C12.2&dist=25&loc=01581&lat=42.2638905&lng=-71.6080009

21st Century Cures Act: https://www.opennotes.org/onc-federal-rule/ Beginning **April 5, 2021,** the program rule on Interoperability, Information Blocking, and ONC Health IT Certification, which implements the 21st Century Cures Act, requires that healthcare providers give patients access without charge to all the health information in their electronic medical records "without delay."

Visiting three hospitals: Onsite visits allow you to experience the hospital in general — the building's age, overall condition, and even how you are treated at the reception desk and by the staff. Once you decide on three to investigate, you should mentally and physically prepare for their process and questions at each hospital related to your illness, even if the questions are redundant. You must understand that you will be working under the orders of their medical professionals at each hospital. You may have to endure a process that can include blood tests, X-rays, MRIs, and CT scans three separate times at three different hospitals.

After the first consultation with the surgeon and their team, X-ray pictures must be taken, and a chemical analysis of your blood must be done. Once you review the tests, more detailed views of the area may be ordered, such as an MRI or CT scan. Each illness will come with its own set of pretesting before the second or third consultation. Although this process can be intrusive or painful, you need to work with the surgeons, specialists, and infectious disease doctors to pinpoint the cause of your ill health and decide where to get treated.

Process and decision factors: During testing, you can measure a hospital using their equipment and how the personnel treats you during the picture-taking and blood analysis. You are not expected to be an expert on medical equipment, but you can look for things, such as whether the X-ray equipment is up to date. Ask if the equipment moves for pictures at different angles, so you do not have to move multiple times. Should you be at a pain level of 6 to 9, your body manipulation tolerance is exceptionally low. Although the technician will try to get the best views based on the surgeon's orders, body part manipulations can exacerbate the pain, making the process almost unbearable. The visits will allow you to see the difference in the number of manipulations and views taken. I feel a hospital with less manipulation has up-to-date equipment. The sight of the equipment at each hospital also may be different. You should be able to see the difference between older equipment and new. You and your advocate should note this by asking, "How dated is this equipment"?

The diagnosis may require MRIs. "This technology is important because MRI scans illustrate more clearly than ever before the difference between healthy and diseased tissue and can provide important information about the brain, spine, joints, and internal organs. It can lead to early detection and treatment of disease and has no known side effects." (Saint Michaels Hospital)

Do not be concerned if an outside organization takes the MRI. It will not affect what the doctors see. However, the hospital owning MRI equipment may show the hospital's dedication to investing money into the best possible diagnoses.

CT scans are usually the third picture ordered by a specialist. According to Mercycare, "CT scans are a valuable diagnostic tool. They can detect some conditions that conventional X-rays cannot because CT scans can show a 3D view of the body's section being studied. CT scans are also useful for monitoring a patient's progress during or after treatment."

Using the CT scan, your specialist can inspect the size, shape, texture, and overall health of your body's internal structures. They can use these images to get relevant data about your health, including the location, extent, and severity of any maladies you may have, like a blockage in your heart." (www.mercycare.org)

There are *risks* to the CT scans, so discuss them with the doctor. In Kim O'Brien's case, the benefits far outweighed the risks. According to www.patientinfo.org, "CT scans of the brain can be affected by bone nearby. High doses of radiation are involved in CT scanning – a chest CT scan is equivalent to 350 chest X-rays, CT abdomen to 400 chest X-rays, and CT pulmonary angiography 750 chest X-rays."

Onsite walkthrough: Although testing processes are diverse, they all have the following categories in common, which you and your advocate can investigate during your consultations and picture-taking.

Staff: The staff set the culture of the recovery wings. You should ask if the RN, CNA, and PNA overlap in their responsibilities. A team effort on any floor provides you with cooperative support for immediate needs such as bathroom trips, answering the call button, body adjustments, and much more.

Room after the surgery: You and your advocate should notice the size of the room – one or two beds, bathroom (just one or do you share with another patient?), TV, menus, and call button location. Depending on your illness and surgery, movement may be restricted and limited so that privacy could be a topic on your checklist. During my stays after operations, the distinction between the orthopedic rooms at the hospital on the South Coast and outside Boston was night and day.

Cleanliness: Infections are more likely to occur during an operation, and the first reduce the probability that you will contract an inflection. It would be best if you looked for a clean/spotless bathroom and bed area. The floor, the tools surrounding the sleeping area, and the bed itself must be sterile. During your walkthrough, see if the staff are using gloves and sterilizing their hands while performing tasks. The staff's garments and uniforms must be clean.

Onsite physical therapists: The new and improved recovery method involves getting you out of bed and walking as soon after surgery as possible, using tools, if necessary. The tools could be a walker, wheelchair, crutches, or simply independently moving legs and arms. Nurses and assistants can ensure that this happens but working with an onsite physical therapist (PT) is far better. The PT will know safe techniques for movement while measuring your baseline ability. The physical therapists work within your abilities and reinforce daily improvements until you are discharged to a home or a rehabilitation facility.

Records: You should ask how you can acquire all current records, how long it takes to receive them, and if paperwork authorizing records release is needed. *It is your right to ask and receive all reports, X-rays, and scans!* You want the hospital to release the reports without objection. It is your legal right under HIPAA.

Food and meals: A fast recovery requires excellent food. You should ask to look at the primary menu and a secondary menu if they have one. Look for versatility and the frequency food and drinks can be ordered and are delivered. Good food makes the post-operation tolerable.

Selecting a surgeon

Validation of the diagnosis: A diagnosis should not be valid until you have done due diligence by having multiple specialists pinpoint the problem. That is why we must know the medical professionals' obligations to the patient. At every phase of a potentially deadly diagnosis, we have the right to ask the difficult questions. Any pre-operational interviews will assist in the decisions and help improve your self-confidence and trust in medical professionals and the quality of their teams.

You must decide on the best surgeon. That statement may seem like common sense or even elementary, yet more people only engage with surgeons referred to them by their primary doctors, who may work with the same HMO, or by family members or friends. Some general practitioners or primary care doctors might not know more about a surgeon than what the hospital or HMO tells them.

No matter what decision you make, get a second and even third opinion. This will reduce your feelings of fear and apprehension. If they all have a similar diagnosis, you have confirmed the illness and eliminated doubts that might be running through your mind. In addition, their opinions and suggested processes may all match, which is a great stress reliever.

Lea, the registered nurse from Boston, said, "Get not only different opinions but also research both the hospitals and the surgeons. Check with the Joint Commission and watch for deficiencies. Go online and check their credentials, and most of all, ask questions."

Here are actual accounts of patients who did not acquire additional opinions.

- I was at a Level 5 to 6 on the pain scale. I followed my primary's referral and went to a spine specialist. After X-rays and an MRI, I was told my spinal disks were touching the sciatic nerves. The corrective surgery plan was to shave the disks, relieving pressure on the nerves. The result was an infection, which led to three more operations, induced comas, and blood transfusions. The damage had been done, and I was diagnosed as a disabled person. Years later, I received the reports of the operation. During the third operation, the surgical team was still removing bone chips from the first operation."

Do you see my mistakes? I did not investigate other hospitals and surgeons with the process you are reading about. I did not ask for the reports after I was taken off life support. Those reports would have let me know the truth of what happened and dictated any legal decisions.

- I met Dan K. at a football playoff party. The doctors told him that the disks in his lower spine had lost cartilage, and the disks had to be fused. The procedure required screws to hold the disks together. After the operation and during recovery at a hospital outside of Worcester, Massachusetts, the surgical team discovered that the tip of the screw went too far into the spine. The lead surgeon and his team confirmed the unfortunate damage and that further surgery could never reverse the mistake. To this day, Dan carries a picture of the MRI and the surgeon's name on his phone; he also walks with a limp.

Neither Dan nor I got a second opinion or visited another hospital. Yet, we both could have prevented a botched operation.

Investigate experience: Let us look at some essential definitions.

Definition of a surgeon: "a medical specialist who practices surgery."

Definition of specialist: "one who specializes in a particular occupation, practice, or field of study" (American College of Surgeons)

"The specialist surgeon must study medicine as an undergraduate, then at a medical school for four years of study. In the fourth year, the individual earns a residency at a hospital for hands-on training. The residency could last three to seven years, depending on the specialty the doctor has chosen. The doctors may then enter their own practice by achieving the specialty status." (American College of Surgeons)

The American College of Surgeons recognizes fourteen surgical specialties:

- cardiothoracic surgery
- colon and rectal surgery
- general surgery
- gynecology and obstetrics
- gynecologic oncology
- neurological surgery
- ophthalmic surgery
- oral and maxillofacial surgery
- orthopedic surgery
- otorhinolaryngology
- pediatric surgery
- plastic and maxillofacial surgery
- urology
- vascular surgery

Within those fourteen surgical specialty titles, there are subsets in which doctors can specialize even more. For example, one doctor works only on "hands," and another doctor works only on "hips and knees"; both fall under orthopedic medicine.

I had four spinal operations, one knee operation, and six hip/joint operations. The spine specialist had his specialty, while the joint surgeons had their specialty. When confronting a surgeon during the interview process, make sure you know to whom you are talking. Be sure to research the doctor's specialty, the dangers of the operation, questions to ask, and the operation's benefits. If the doctor is vague or defensive when you ask your questions, you should consult another specialist.

Doctors go through many years of intensive study, hands-on work, supervision, and more learning based on their specialties. Questions help in choosing a doctor you are comfortable with to heal your diagnosed condition.

American Board of Medical Specialists (ABMS) is another resource to find a specialist and validate their credentials. (www.abms.org)

The ABMS website contains data on specific specialties, the doctors associated with a specialty, and where you can find them. In addition, their website states: "Service for Patients and Their Families – When selecting physicians, it's wise to invest some time and energy in learning more about their skills and training, as well as the quality of care they provide. Consider several sources of information, including whether the physician is board-certified and meets the requirements of the ABMS Program for Maintenance of Certification (ABMS MOC®) to learn the board certification status of physicians, including whether they are meeting the obligations of an ABMS Member Board MOC program.

Compensation of the specialist: The specialist's justification and validation for compensation are based on their extended training. On page 39 of *Prescription for Bankruptcy — A doctor's perspective of a failing healthcare system and how we can fix it,* Doctor Edward Hoffer wrote, "Doctors undergo a long period of education and post-graduate training, and often work under stressful conditions. They are entitled to be paid comparably to professionals who perform similarly highly skilled work."

On page 12, Doctor Hoffer wrote, "American physicians earn approximately double what doctors earn in Europe. In 2017, a salary survey found that US doctors earned an average of $294,000 annually. Primary care physicians average $212,000 and specialists $316,000."

Due to the amount of time, cost of extensive training, and stressful conditions of their work, you can feel comfortable that the higher level of compensation can be relative to the training and experience of the specialist you chose.

Questions and answers: As a patient with a diagnosed illness, it is your right to ask questions of any medical professional you encounter. Question-and-answer sessions with the surgeon are critical to developing a good relationship and level of comfort and rapport. You and your advocate should listen carefully and document every consultation.

This method will help you recognize any inconsistency among the surgeons at the three hospitals you visit. However, should the answers and diagnosis be the same, then you have done your best self-advocacy. Ideally, you need at least two surgeons' reports with the same diagnosis. At that point, the decision becomes which hospital and which surgeon.

If you have the time to research the process, ask the doctors for the name of the illness and the corrective procedure. You can personally investigate the diagnosis, the names of the process the surgeon will use, and its risks. For example, after my last hip was in place, I could have Googled "probability of living after a dual revision of infected hips." I later found a study of the issue from PMC — National Institute of Health — Lorenzo Fagotti and others. The survival rate was 76 percent, which is much better than I was led to believe.

The information you get before the operation should provide more intelligent questions for you to ask the surgeons and their team.

Questions to ask include:

- Length of time at the hospital?
- How many years focusing on a specialty?
- Teaming up with another experienced surgeon?
- Using residents during the operation, and what is their role?

    Are they just observing?
    Are they opening and closing?

What year of residency and experience do they have?

- What process will the surgical team use?
- Current sterilization process for the operating theater before surgeries scheduled daily? Between surgeries?

  These examples are orthopedic questions.

  - Are they planning on operating on the hip from the anterior or posterior? Why?
  - Is the surgical team using a hands-on scalpel approach or a Robotic-Arm Assisted Surgery? You can use both styles for joint conditions.
  - Will the medical team leave the wound open for a period after the surgery? Are drains used?
  - Will rehabilitation be needed after surgery? Should it be home therapy, outpatient therapy, or at a rehabilitation facility?

- Should there be multiple operations, what to expect between operations?
- After one of the multiple operations, what to expect in quality of life? Examples: effect on the senses, ability to walk, ability to talk, long-term need for mobility tools, pain levels, scar tissue repercussions, and what medications and for how long?
- If the operation(s) is(are) not successful, what is expected to happen?

These questions were provided by Lea, a head registered nurse in Boston, and are from "Ask Your Physician, Agency for Health Research":

Diagnosis

- What is my disease/condition called?
- How can I expect to feel?
- How long am I likely to feel this way?
- Will I need any tests or procedures? If so, what are they? Are they done in the doctor's office or at another facility? Is the test/ procedure done at a hospital? Will it be done on an outpatient basis, or will I need to stay at the hospital? What answers could the test/procedure provide?

Treatment:

- What treatment do you recommend (surgery, medication, dietary change, exercise, therapy)?
- What results do you expect from this treatment (such as pain relief, cure)?
- Are there alternatives to the treatment? (Ask for recommended alternative medications, lifestyle changes, for example)?
- Will over-the-counter medications, herbs, or supplements interfere or interact with the medicine you are prescribing?

Medication:

- What are the generic and brand names of all my medications?
- How and when should I take it (time or how often; with or without food; for how long)?
- What do I need to know about the other medications I take?
- What should these medications do for me (cure an infection, relieve pain or inflammation)?
- What side effects might I encounter, and do they go away?

Doctor Edward Hoffer, in his book *Prescription for Bankruptcy*, suggests asking the following questions of any doctor you are considering:

- Why did you conclude that I have this condition — on what basis?
- What else could it be, and have you conclusively ruled out other conditions?
- How do you plan to be sure? Do I need other tests or opinions?
- If we are treating this new condition, when should I see improvement? When should I call or come in if I do not improve?

Answers: There are distinct similarities in selecting and working with surgeons. One similarity is that each surgeon gets right to the issues to be discussed, what you have, and what they can do or cannot do. The surgeon and staff who have read all the images and reports are in an expert position and can take the lead on your care while you are attached to their office. Expect open and frank conversations at each consultation with the doctor. Include the medical team when appropriate.

Note: If the surgeon and team have not viewed the pictures and read the reports, cross that surgeon off the list.

Do not expect that the surgeon will converse about family, friends, or other doctors. They know what they are doing, they have many patients waiting, and they schedule full days for operations during the week, so time is significant.

Nonverbal answers that are useful: Consistency of opinions the team present, level of confidence of the surgeon, inflection in the voice, body movements, and notes taken by the advocate about the consultation for future reference.

These are ways to measure the consultation:

- Consistency in the diagnosis of at least two surgeons.
- If there is a surgical team, all members should be present.
- Inflection in the voice and body movements. This is very subjective, so I would suggest bringing in a second person and/or advocate to listen to the conversation. If the surgeon does not want to do the work or is not confident, you both will be able to recognize it. The same holds for the voice. You should hear the confidence of the doctor and the team, eye contact,

using your hands to discuss the images, and the way the surgeon greets you.

- An advocate taking notes during a consultation will write down the surgeon's answers. The patient asks the questions, and the advocate takes the notes. An advocate improves concentration during a consultation, monitors consistency, and records detailed solutions to the questions. The advocate may provide questions during a consultation.

K. O'Brien took her primary doctor's advice and went to the neurologist she suggested. The first neurological specialist diagnosed Kim O'Brien with severe degeneration in the cervical disc C 5–6 and C 6–7. After that, the specialist referred her to several orthopedic surgeons and neurosurgeons. There were no answers, just assumptions by the doctors.

K Obrien wrote: "I began setting up appointments with these doctors to gather opinions. The first stop was to the orthopedic surgeon. I just was not impressed with his flippant attitude once he heard my pain levels were low. The second appointment was with a neurosurgeon that my brother-in-law went to for a lower back fusion. He was nice and looked over all the information I had, and he also said he would wait to do surgery as my symptoms were 'mild' along with my pain levels. At that point, I decided that I would wait a few weeks to see how I was feeling. I felt defeated. I am the one walking around feeling dizzy and numb all the time, but two doctors told me they would wait to do surgery."

The importance of understanding Diagnosis-Related Groups (DRGs): Once the surgeons have made their diagnosis and the surgeon's recommendation has been made, ask the question:

- Ask the doctor what Diagnosis-Related Group is your staff assigning me on the hospital form for admission?

This question is directly tied to what the surgeon feels is the level of care you need from the hospital, the length of time you can be in the hospital, and insurance payments to the hospital and the surgeon.

- What Diagnosis-Related Group code is the staff in medical recordings providing to the hospital and rehabilitation facilities for my condition and surgery?

"DRGs are a means of classifying a patient under a group where those assigned are likely to need a similar level of hospital resources for their care. ... The system was to be used to help hospital administrators control physician behavior." Vincari Media, February 7, 2013

Carevoyance.com says, "DRGs allow the healthcare provider to provide more information on the severity of the patient's illness within the group and CMS (Centers for Medicare and Medicaid Services for health coverages) to adjust costs based on different stages in the progression of an illness or complications or comorbidities (CCs)." The DRG codes entered in the system by the surgeon and staff determine a minimum and maximum insurance coverage.

The DRG's importance is explained in an article by Michael Damrich in *General Surgery News* (February 2013), "What is a Diagnosis-Related Group and Why You Should Care?":

"Diagnosis-Related Groups (DRGs) are a means of classifying a patient under a group where those assigned are likely to need a similar hospital resources level for their care. This allows hospital administrators to more accurately determine the type of resources needed to treat a group and predict the cost of that treatment more closely."

"Deciding on the most appropriate DRG level to assign a patient is determined by several factors, including the International Classification of Diseases (ICD) code or codes recorded during hospital admission. There are generally three major disease categories, with a higher weight given for more serious illnesses. ICD diagnoses are assigned to one of three categories: neutral, comorbid condition (CC), or major comorbid condition (MCC). Documentation of an MCC condition will trigger the highest DRG level for that condition. For example, if when performing an appendectomy, a physician simply records the diagnosis as "appendicitis," the lowest or neutral DRG category will be applied. Recording the condition as "acute appendicitis" means that the CC category will be applied. An abscess or peritonitis falls under the MCC category, the highest level of DRG assignment, and patient care resources.

"The same system is being used to judge the quality of care that a physician delivers. Because each admission or procedure is attributed to an individual physician, physicians are given a score based on the severity of a patient's documented illness. If the documentation is nonspecific, this forms the assumption that a patient has fewer morbidities, costs less to care for, and requires a shorter hospital length of stay. Physicians who maintain more accurate documentation procedures will fare better than those who may provide equal quality of care but do not document."

"The hospital will be paid one lump sum for your stay and surgery. The correct code correlates to your maximum quality of care. Should there be a misdiagnosis and you must be readmitted, insurance could be at risk and negatively affects the hospital's Joint Commission credentials."

Websites to help your search and verification:

www.checkbook.org has data about selecting the best doctors and other providers to make decisions about your medical care.

www.abms.org; The American Board of Medical Specialties (ABMS) is an independent, not-for-profit organization founded in 1933 to set professional standards for physician practice and board certification.

https://www.medicare.gov/physiciancompare/ The Medicare website for finding a surgeon and comparing surgeons.

https://www.opennotes.org/onc-federal-rule/ **Federal Rules Mandating Open Notes**: On April 5, 2021, federal rules implemented the bipartisan 21st Century Cures Act specifying that eight types of clinical notes are among electronic information that must not be blocked and must be made available free of charge to patients. To meet the interests of some patients, the rules allow specified exceptions.

Roles of medical professionals and the patient perspective

A surgeon's role and patient perspective: The American College of Surgeons (ACS) says: "Although the workplace settings may vary, one factor remains the same: The surgical profession is one of responsibility and leadership. The surgeon is responsible for the patient's preoperative diagnosis, operating, and providing the patient with post-operative surgical care and treatment. The surgeon is also looked upon as the leader of the surgical team."

I asked a kidney specialist at Lahey Hospital in Lexington, Massachusetts, what he sees his role as. The response mirrored the ACS definition: "I look at my practice as Diagnosis – Partnership – Therapy." His input validates the formal definition of partnership. It reflects respect for the patient. He relies on the patient to be cooperative and work as part of the team. Included in the concept of "partnership" will be the operation. At this point, the patient must be committed to the procedures and therapy to follow.

Due to the difficulty of a double revision of my hips, the surgeon had to be a leader. *My choice was based on his reputation and skill, but also his role as a leader. As I understood the* *team's personalities, it was imperative to adjust to each team member's perspective of what needed to be done and how to do it. For example, before and after each operation, my lead surgeon would step into my holding area for a preoperative checkup. Just by knowing his way with a patient, I knew he was testing my attitude before being wheeled into the operating room by asking me how I was. I ended each last-minute visit with, "I am ready; let's get it done!" That was when the lead surgeon would smile.*

As a leader, the surgeon's control extends to therapy and recommendation for rehabilitation. Whether doctor's instructions pertain to therapy, release to home care, time at a skilled nursing rehabilitation facility or referral to an acute rehabilitation facility, the medical professional's orders must be followed. At this point, you can ask questions and provide input. The surgeon's responsibility is to listen to your perspective, give an answer, and make changes as necessary.

The patient's perspective: The patients I have spoken with said they wanted the doctor to visit before and after the operation. When the surgeon visits after the operation, you can ask more questions and hear how the procedure went from the surgeon's perspective. The surgeon, at that time, is still your doctor. They are in control and lead.

Kim's journey took her to a fourth opinion because her symptoms were alarming, yet the pain was mild. A lead surgeon listened and used technology when the others did not. She was astute enough to have asked the previous specialists for their reports and brought those reports and MRIs with her for her last opinion.

She states, "One day, I was at work, and both my legs went completely numb. I felt like I could barely walk. I decided that was it! I was headed to the last neurosurgeon on my list. I made the appointment and went in the next week. This man walked into the appointment, listened to everything I said, looked at the MRI with me, and decided that we needed to order a CT scan because he believed there was more to 'the story.' Well, he was right. The scan showed that I had a large bone spur compressing my spinal cord. The compression was the cause of many of my symptoms, and he wanted to do surgery as soon as possible. Two weeks later, I had my spinal fusion with complete success, and pain levels right after the surgery were very mild.

"This doctor was amazing. He was extremely laid back, patient, and kind. He made me feel like I knew what I was talking about and took what I said seriously. Before my appointment, I checked his credentials, and he received his medical degree at Princeton University. That was more than impressive to me. I would rate my experience with this neurosurgeon as exceptional.

I am five years out from the surgery and have experienced no pain or symptoms of any kind. I am glad that I 'shopped around' before I took the word of just one doctor. I learned a valuable lesson from watching my best friend suffer through the same surgery two years before mine. She had the surgery done with the same orthopedist I first went to see, and she has not had the success I have had. She told me multiple times that she wished she got more than one opinion. She will be headed back into surgery within the next six months. This time she will be going with my neurosurgeon and is hoping for a better outcome." – K. O'Brien.

The previous diagnoses were incorrect, and additional tests had not been made. Pain levels and not the symptoms described by O'Brien's misdirected the previous specialists. The fantastic facts are that she continued to pursue additional opinions and checked the surgeon's credentials. The role of the primary doctor concerning the specialist is to investigate multiple variables and then eliminate the variables that do not apply. Her earlier surgeons did not do this. They forgot their role.

The rehabilitation facility doctor's role: Brainline.org defines floor rehabilitation doctors as "rehabilitation (PM&R) physicians, also known as physiatrists, treating a wide variety of medical conditions affecting the brain, spinal cord, nerves, bones, joints, ligaments, muscles, and tendons. Specifically, PM&R physicians: Treat patients of all ages. Focus treatment on function."

The American Academy of Physical Medicine and Rehabilitation says: "Physiatrists maximize what a patient can do and assist the patient in adapting to what he or she cannot. A physiatrist should be consulted when pain, weakness, or disability is preventing a patient from achieving their desired level of independence."

Each rehabilitation facility must have a rehabilitation doctor to carry on what the surgeons have diagnosed and their prescribed treatment. You might say the surgeons "pass the baton to the physiatrist." The physiatrist has read the operation notes, has reviewed the medications, and may prescribe a new medicine. The rehabilitation doctor will now be the go-to physician for any variations from the standard specialty illness while at the rehabilitation facility. Should there be any health variations, the floor doctor is the medical professional to be informed immediately.

As you progress through rehabilitation, other departments will take charge, and the physiatrist will rarely be seen until discharge. Each physiatrist has a reasonably large number of patients under their care, and those patients rotate in and out of rehabilitation constantly. Therefore, these doctors must focus on any acute issues that arise in patients at a rehabilitation facility.

The patient's perspective: Watch and learn about the medical professionals at the rehabilitation facility. If you are being mistreated, perceive complications, or request a formal status report, you must notify the doctor in charge. In addition, you should let your advocate know of any situation that affects your safety. If necessary, be your advocate and go to the top.

During twelve stays at each rehabilitation facility, I rarely interacted with the physiatrist other than saying hello while passing in the hallways. When my medicine had not been issued, or the correct amount was wrong, I notified the head nurse and the doctor. During most of my stays at rehabilitation facilities, I had no official advocate, so self-advocacy was necessary for my safety for years.

The physician assistant's role: Second to the rigorous education and training, a surgical specialist must undergo the physician assistant (PA) must also have special medical training. Many people have never heard of PAs. However, when a PA is assigned to a patient in the hospital, acute care rehabilitation, or subacute rehabilitation, they have earned the same respect as the physician. The PA works with a doctor on the floor or has the expertise to work independently.

The Get Educated website says: "Physician Assistants (PA) are medical professionals who diagnose illness; develop and manage treatment plans; prescribe medications; and often serve as a patient's principal caregiver."
(www.geteducated.com)

"In most cases, a physician assistant will need a master's degree from an accredited institution (two years of post-graduate education after completing a four-year degree). Essentially, you're looking at six years of rigorous education in total to become a physician assistant."
(www.geteducated.com)

The training and education: "[P]physician assistants (PAs) must complete a PA graduate program accredited by the **Accreditation Review Commission on Education for the**

Physician Assistant. Accredited graduate degree programs include classroom instruction, lab instruction, and clinical rotations. Most programs are about 26 months in duration and include at least 2,000 hours of clinical rotations."
(www.arc-pa.org)

The physician assistant must learn concepts of person-centered care, transitions of care, discharge planning, comprehensive assessment for rehabilitation, mobility management, ethics, end-of-life care, nursing home care, and best practices for addressing syndromes (a group of symptoms).

I do not believe the physician assistant has to be in your interview process. Knowing they are on the floor and available is comfortable enough. The doctor may be hard to find after surgery, but you have another medical professional leader consulting and supporting you *if* the organization has hired a PA.

Out of the twelve rehabilitation facilities, only three had a PA on staff. While volunteering at a rehabilitation facility, I saw a young woman with a stethoscope around her neck holding a patient's chart. She interrupted my work with a patient, so I asked who she was. She let me know with no smile on her face. It was then I learned that the physician assistant had authority and deserved respect.

To reduce any confusion, we must understand the difference between a physician's assistant and a nurse practitioner: "On a fundamental level, a nurse practitioner attends a nursing school while a physician's assistant attends a medical school

or center of medicine. ... Physician Assistants follow a disease-centered model, in which they focus on the biologic and pathologic components of health, and practice assessment, diagnosis, and treatment."
(www.nursepractitionerschools.com, February 14, 2020)

The patient's perspective: Though the physician's assistant can be seen from a different perspective as a doctor, the PA demands the same respect. The patient must also perform the same due diligence if the doctor in charge relies highly on the PA for assistance. Diagnosis and confirmation with other opinions are just as crucial as opinion confirmation with the doctor should the PA accept that role.

The nurse practitioner's role: The definition of a nurse practitioner, from Nurse Practitioner School, is "a nurse who is qualified to treat certain medical conditions without the direct supervision of a doctor."

My multiple operations and rehabilitation visits allowed me the privilege to meet and be seen by at least eight nurse practitioners. These medical professionals, in my case, were the link to the primary and specialty surgical doctors. These men and women have studied and trained by nurse specialty schools at the physician's level. Therefore, the NP's diagnosis and examinations should be taken seriously and with respect. Yes, they carry stethoscopes. Here are statements from Lexico Dictionary that will help you better understand:

> "A nurse practitioner performs a preoperative history and physical examination."

"Each practice employed a nurse who had completed a one- or two-year nurse practitioner training program with a diploma at BSc or MSc level."

"Patients have come to accept seeing a nurse practitioner in place of a physician for routine checkups and office visits."

The patient's perspective: At the first meeting after an operation, I met with Dr. Henderson and the nurse practitioner when I was diagnosed with multiple hip infections. In my mind, it was time to know the process to be used to clear the infections, so I asked the question to Dr. Henderson's nurse practitioner. Her response was, "Bill, this is an exceedingly rare case, and we are making it up as we go along." The surgeon later told me, "We are working in the dark!" My perception was that the nurse practitioner was in sync with the surgeon; their responses were consistent. In addition, she was now my point person since the surgeon was busy with other surgeries.

In 2021, since the hip infections were cleared up and pain reduced, I decided to have another opinion on the condition of my spine. What state was it in, and what to expect? The surgeons who operated on my hips had now moved to Lahey Hospital and Medical Center, so I decided to have Lahey's Neurosurgery department provide the new opinion.

I was introduced to Kimberly A., a Nurse Practitioner, MSN, NP-C, for the preliminary examination and next steps. After an MRI, I met with her for the follow-up consultation. Kimberly went through my spinal issues in great detail after reviewing my MRI and records. So much so that I now understood what went wrong in 2011 and what corrections could be done, which were none. But she did have hope for some injections, which may or may not work; at least she gave me hope since I can only walk 50 yards before pain stops me and I must rest. I asked Kimberly how she liked being a Nurse Practitioner. Her response was, "I love every minute of it. I take the work and my patients very seriously. This is a great place to work." She reminded me of the kidney specialist and his attitude toward his profession.

The registered nurse's role: The description of the registered nursing role is, "a registered nurse (RN) job includes monitoring, recording, and reporting symptoms or changes in patients' conditions. They are tasked with maintaining accurate patient reports and medical histories, administering medication and treatment to patients, and observing reactions or side effects." (thebalancecareers.com)

There is always a nurse's station on each hospital or facility floor, and it is a must that you learn who the head nurse and floor nurses are during each shift. These medical professionals have earned their titles and their jobs, but events can happen that make you feel uncomfortable or neglected. This is the time action that should be taken by you or your advocate to report the events to the head nurse or directors. The directors and the head nurse should take action to correct the issues. I address this again in the "warning signs" section of the book.

By working well with the registered nurse, you have achieved the right to ask questions at any time, but do not overdo the privilege.

One registered nurse's role is to check the wound, change the bandages, and report your daily status in the computer system. Should you have a wound from surgery that required stitches, the RN may be the person to remove the stitches if the surgeon or facility's doctor has assigned the RN that responsibility.

Positive interaction between you and the registered nurse is imperative. Standard procedures, such as changing the dressing or delivering medication at the right time, require both a good rapport and a common goal for recovery. For example, do both parties agree that the process was done correctly? One suggestion is to ask another registered nurse from another shift to look at the dressing.

During one of my interviews with Brian Masters, he told me it was a daily procedure to have his wound checked and rewrapped. During the process, the first nurse used gauze as the first layer of the wrap. Everything looked fine, so she applied a second wrap with a tight cloth, covering the gauze. Using gauze for a wound that contains stitches protruding from the skin is not the best procedure.

When Brian became more active, the itching increased, the wrap became loose, and blood started to reappear, so he asked the nurse to look at the wound. The second nurse removed the second layer, and the gauze layer started to appear. It was apparent that the gauze had wrapped around the stitches from the wound. Not only was there incredible pain in removing the gauze, removing the wrap loosened the stitches. He had to undergo blood cleaning, sterilizing the incision, replacing the loose stitches, and rewrapping the incision.

The only benefit of the mistake was that the head nurse took the time to retrain her staff on the use of gauze for wounds.

You need to contact the registered nurse as soon as possible if you feel pain, are uncomfortable, feel ill, or have signs of a problem, like leakage of blood. You must be aware that a nurse's time on the floor is precious. They have a patient ratio to nurse of 5 to 1, 6 to 1, or as high as 8 to 1. They are responsible for reporting each visit, recording what was discussed, acting, and ordering medicines. It is a time-consuming process, so be considerate.

The patient's perspective: *In my opinion, the nurses working in the post-operation hospital and acute care and subacute care (post-acute care) are angels of mercy. That old statement still holds today. I use the saying, "It is not a doctor who saves the patient. It is* the nurses."

The actual stories I am about to relate will reinforce suggested behaviors and how to work with the nurses. I also include unfortunate episodes and stories to illustrate awareness and recommended action.

Some individuals describe a registered nurse as an angel of mercy. Brian M., who wrote *Road to Addiction – Highways to Recovery,* tells a story of just such a nurse. Brian had stayed in the hospital for three days, the number of days necessary to get insurance coverage (Medicare) and a rehabilitation facility recommendation. Before leaving his bed at the hospital, Brian asked the nurse if she had sent his prescriptions to the skilled nursing rehabilitation (post-acute) facility. The nurse, of two months, responded, "As you can see, we are extremely busy." Brian let it go. Brian wrote:

> "**An angel of mercy:** After being sent to the rehabilitation facility, I settled into the bed and the normal parade of staff came to introduce themselves; the room nurses, the floor nurse, and the orderly. Hours later, I called the nurse because the pain increased. The nurse on duty explained to me that the prescriptions had not been transferred from the hospital to the facility's doctor." Since it was after hours and no one in either facility was available, pain medication could not be given to him. Brian did the math and realized that meant 18 hours after a total hip replacement operation; he would have *no* medication of any kind, not even aspirin. The result was him screaming in pain.
>
> The nursing and staff shift changed, and the night staff came on duty. He looked up, and an older nurse was standing above him, holding a small cup with two pills and a cup of water. She smiled and asked Brian to take the pills. Without hesitation, the meds went down his throat as fast as he could swallow. The nurse said, "I have no comments about why this was not addressed, but I have been a nurse all my life. We must use common sense. I gave you two Tylenol with codeine. That should help until morning."

The truth is that a rehabilitation facility should have an Emergency Drug Box (EDB), which is kept next to the "crash cart." It holds medication, such as pain killers, as a backup for such emergencies. The nurses must call the facility's doctor and get the authority to give the medicine to the patient, which the day staff did not do in this case. The fact is that the EDB exists. At a time like this, it is vital to be your advocate or call your advocate.

Medication neglect: Regrettably, there are times the nurse is not delivering pain medicine on time. If your medication is delayed when it should be delivered, you will have an additional hour of pain. I have interviewed patients on this topic, and they received comments from the RN, such as, "I am going down to each room, and when I get to your room, you will have it." In other situations, they did not respond at all.

Attempting to correct the problem by sitting next to the medication cart backfires typically. The result of subtly going into the hallway and distracting the nurse could be, "You're not going to get what you need" or "You're not my favorite patient."

A solution to the problem is a computer system that tracks when the nurses dispense medicines. In addition, the med cart will have a mobile computer to input times and notes for the audit trail.

Nelsa, the nursing director at one of the best rehabilitation facilities I stayed at, enlightened me about their software and process. She told me, "Should a nurse be consistently late with meds, the system will show it via the computer screen or on paper. The system will tell us when the med should be delivered and when it was delivered. The director of nursing or the nurse in charge of the floor can address any problem. Should a patient receive medication late or have another issue, the patient should go to the head of nursing for an explanation and help."

Lea, an RN at a leading hospital in Boston, used a prepackaged medicine packets system. She said, "It is an older system, but it worked. If any of a patient's medicine is still in the daily packet, then a mistake has been made, and there will be a floor audit at the end of the shift."

This is another question for the rehabilitation facility interview: Do they have either system or any system at all?

Should similar events continue to happen, it is your responsibility to either call your advocate or be your advocate. If a medication is an hour late, it has affected your hours of pain. For example, if the medicine is to be given every four hours and the medication is an hour late, you have five hours of pain. Now you must wait another four hours for your next medicine. If this nurse's lateness continues at the following application, you have gained another hour of pain.

There is always the nurse who follows their role to the letter and beyond the call of duty. While staying at a facility just outside of Worcester, Massachusetts, a nurse named Alexa worked with me professionally, with spirit and emotion.

Whether using the lift to elevate a patient in and out of bed or just checking blood pressure, she did it with a smile. When the orders indicated that medicine was to be delivered, she was right on time.

The certified nursing assistant (CNA) role: According to US LEGAL, a "Certified nursing assistant (CNA) is a person who assists patients with healthcare needs and cares for a patient who is ill or recovering from a surgery or disease. A registered professional nurse assigns CNA duty. Sometimes they provide service on daily living activities [and] bedside care, including basic nursing procedures under the supervision of a registered nurse."

The definition is technically correct, but it does not emphasize the great need for the CNA. The CNA is the conduit between you and the nursing staff. They are the front line in your care, whether you are recovering from an operation, being evaluated for long-term care, or in permanent long-term care.

Should issues occur outside the CNA's definition of duties and medical knowledge, the nurse on duty (for that patient, in that wing) should be called. If the nurse is busy with urgent care, the head nurse or RN at the nurse's station must be aware of the situation. Events outside CNA duties are blood loss, abnormal behaviors such as seizures, a patient falling, increases in temperature, or the patient wandering or continually getting out of bed.

Before going into the hospital, rehabilitation facility, or nursing home, you and your advocate need to know the CNAs and the ratio of CNA to the number of patients.

> **Responsibilities that count:** Answering the room light in the hallway, emptying the urinal bottles and bedpans, enforcing the no-wandering orders, making sure you do not go into the bathroom unescorted (this important if you are using a walker or wheelchair), use of gait belts, guiding you in and out of the wheelchair, escorting and setting up bathing are just a few activities that CNAs perform.

A gait belt is for your safety and is a precious tool for good patient care. The use of gait belts may be embarrassing or humiliating to you, but the risk of falling increases dramatically without them. The result could be damaged implants or stitches, or a broken foot, knee, arm, or hip. A concussion from falling could send you back to the hospital to begin rehabilitation all over again. Being disagreeable and impatient may lead to painful outcomes if you do not adhere to orders and let the gait belt be put on you.

Professional training and experience prepare CNAs for unexpected services that prevent harm to patients in their care.

> **Special service examples:** Washing hands and wearing gloves to reduce infections, making changes in the bed being used, implementing pain management standards of practice, delivering effective and pleasant communication, and ordering food before the cafeteria closes. These special

services mean the difference between a bad rehabilitation experience and a productive stay.

In my experience, CNAs provide care that is not defined in their role, such as the ability to laugh with you, talk to you, and add good cheer while you are in an unfamiliar place or with a person they have only just met.

I loved when the CNA and/or the floor nurse would bring liquid refreshments and/or snacks without being asked.

Emotion and empathy are behaviors required of the CNA in the training manuals, but these are not learned behaviors. Sincere emotion and empathy can be expressed by someone who means well and identifies with the patient. However, organizations cannot train or teach empathy; the delivery of emotion is embedded in a person's personality.

I asked a certified nursing assistant, DA Swanson, what a CNA expects to see from patients in their care, whether in acute or post-acute rehabilitation.

She replied: "I've helped folks in their homes who have been through both of those levels of care. Every patient is different. Acute rehabilitation is shorter and more intense, while post-acute is a long process, which is more likely where I would be helpful. As a CNA, I would watch and listen to a client/patient to assess if they are up to the challenge they are facing. Often folks who are facing rehab have been through that before.

"It could be that they have become discouraged and worn out, and you are there to assist in their next attempt at healing or improvement. As a CNA, I hope to expect a tolerant attitude toward them and a readiness, to begin with, for the assistance I offer. It is not about what I expect from them as much as what they expect from themselves. I am the reminder and support when frustration and fatigue set in. During home care, I would back up a physical therapist and work in the home or the facility to assist a client with daily living post-surgery activities. I have been in both those levels of rehab with hip and knee replacements. The incentive to get better is an improved quality of life.

"There are different types of rehab: physical and emotional. The way I feel about being a CNA and helping folks in rehab is, 'I'll just walk along with you as you get stronger. If you need to lean on me, I am here. If you need to talk, I will listen, and if you fall, I will help you up. We are going to do this together.'"

DA Swanson has a nursing assistant certification of NAC. The State of Washington uses NAC instead of CNA.

The patient's perspective and behavior change: Amazingly, many new and returning patients do not know what the acronym CNA stands for. Having been to many rehabs owned by different companies, I consider the CNA a necessary professional for personal services. One goal of this book is to educate critical behavioral changes for future or returning patients. Simple as it may seem, the call button at all hospitals and care facilities can cause enormous discord between the CNA and the patient. I want to help change and improve this perception of the patients and the professionals.

The call buttons: Once you have settled in your room, you will be shown the call button next to your bed. The call button activates a light outside the room, which signals that the call button has been pushed. This light will indicate to floor staff that you have a need.

The professional staff has told me that one out of five call lights could be a critical/acute need by the patient, but each room light must be taken seriously and answered. Depending on the organization, time limits are in place as a guide for the staff to respond. The nurse training manuals I have read require a staff response in five to ten minutes.

The patients I interviewed and from my experiences, "the times that the 5-minute time frame is met are few and far between. It will be frustrating to you but pushing the call button over and over does little to help. Repeatedly pushing it only adds frustration and unnecessary discord."

The reason there may be a response problem varies from hospital to hospital, center to center, and facility to facility. Here are the typical reasons for delays:

- The nurse and CNA are addressing more urgent problems.
- The nurse or CNA is engaged in lifting a patient, taking blood, cleaning urine or feces, or taking someone to the shower.
- The organization's CNA and floor nurse requirements fall short of possible to handle; 1 to 5 or even a 1 to 8 ratio.

- The light does not work.
- The call-bell cord was unplugged from the wall.
- The patient has a history of using the call bell for no apparent reason.

The CNA availability and the call-bell response are essential questions to ask during the walkthrough.

The critical need for the certified nursing assistant (CNA): At the Westborough facility where I recuperated from my first hip operation, there was only one CAN. Occasionally, he oversaw the entire floor of thirty-six patients. In a room with three other patients, it was an act of survival to befriend the CNA. Without Bob at the Westborough facility, I would not have received attention, conversed, or received better food. But, unfortunately, even though Bob was responsive and had a good heart, he could not effectively do his job when patients were aggressive, demanding and kept pressing the call button.

When I interviewed Dick, the heart patient at Beth Israel Hospital, I asked how he liked the CNAs at the Braintree Rehabilitation Facility. His response was, "Who"? What is a CNA?" Dick gave an honest answer. I know he was concentrating on pain and getting better, and I know the hospital and the rehabilitation facility had CNAs.

Dick's response is one of the reasons for this book. By not knowing the medical professional in person and understanding their job responsibilities, you could misread what a CNA should do for you.

An example of misunderstanding may come from enforcing the out-of-bed policy, assisting you with bathroom duties, and monitoring you in the bathroom. You must understand the role and the CNA's oath to help you. Your recovery experience will be more comfortable by understanding the CNA's role and acknowledging them as professionals.

Physical and occupational therapy: Merriam-Webster's definition of *physical therapy* says that it is "for the preservation, enhancement, or restoration of movement and physical function impaired or threatened by disease, injury, or disability that [uses] therapeutic exercise, physical modalities (such as massage and electrotherapy), assistive devices, and patient education and training."

Merriam-Webster says that *occupational therapy* is "based on engagement in meaningful activities of daily life (such as self-care skills, education, work, or social interaction) to enable or encourage participation in such activities despite impairments or limitations in physical or mental functioning."

Physical therapy (PT) and occupational therapy (OT) are essential processes that must be taken seriously, whether in a rehabilitation facility, at an outside organization, or your home. Therefore, it is valuable to know your insurance PT and OT policies. You should know the length of time you are eligible to receive the services, the total amount covered, the list of insurance companies they work with, and whether insurance will cover in- and outside-facility patient care for both PT and OT.

I wrote that I am not a medical professional, which includes physical and occupational therapy. Therefore, I will not write about the type of therapy that should be used or needed. Instead, we will look at real-life stories, good and bad, so you will be educated about what to look for in therapy departments, the significance of PT, OT, and the consequences without them.

Physical therapy is a curative process where the body repairs itself with exercise and movements in layperson's terms. A professional works with you to understand the strengths and limitations of extremities and the otolaryngology issues you may have relating to the nose, ear, and throat; the ability to hear and speak is part of the practice. PT includes working on mental adjustments if any. The therapists help you to work and acknowledge positive improvements, from admittance to discharge. The critical tasks for success are when you return to the place you live in. We will discuss home care later in the book.

It does not matter if it is your first or fourth operation; surgery could require days, weeks, or months of physical therapy. Feelings of apprehension and fear can come over you at any time. Ideally, you have scrutinized the facility during the pre-surgery walkthrough. When the assigned therapist comes to take you to the department, you must realize that they are your teacher/instructor during this ordeal, not someone to be feared.

Your discharge from a hospital or post-acute care, or acute care facility depends on physical and occupational therapy personnel and their recommended routines. You must be *approved* for discharge through their departments. Your future health care is in their hands.

"Physical therapists in the acute care setting play an important role in the multi-disciplinary discharge planning process. Discharge to the appropriate level of care often is a goal in acute care physical therapy, and therapists routinely make recommendations regarding discharge placement and any continuing therapy services for patients. Due to short average lengths of admission in acute care, patients often need continued physical therapy services after leaving acute care, and therapists may recommend that continued services take place in the home, a skilled nursing facility (SNF), a rehabilitation facility, or an outpatient setting." (U.S. National Library of Medicine).

The patient's perspective: One of the best ways to understand and differentiate PT and OT facilities is through real patient testimonials. These stories exemplify the need for advocacy and visiting a facility before you go to the hospital. An advocate can help by visiting rehabs while you have the operation. I would ask you to look for the PT and OT departments' infrastructure and the staff's demeanor. You must understand that physical therapists have a great deal of responsibility and power in approving your discharge.

Dick Maggio, the heart patient from the Braintree rehabilitation, thought physical therapy and occupational therapy he received were the best. But, he said, "The physical therapy equipment was extensive. I used the treadmill, resistance bike, table, and bed for getting out of a lying-down position, light weights, and half a car so I could practice getting in and out the driver seat."

Learning how to get in and out of a car is extremely important for almost all operations. For example, Dick's acute rehabilitation facility had a mock car. An excellent example of funding by the organization toward quality care. Scrutiny of the facility before admission should be a top priority once the doctor informs you that therapy will be necessary.

Dick told me that occupational therapy had a kitchen so patients could practice how to get around safely. Dick and other patients would cook in their kitchen, using the refrigerator, utensils, and stove to make omelets, pancakes, and soups. The OT bathroom was functional. He would shower, brush his teeth, and use the toilet. Dick was experiencing real-life techniques, equipment, and tools that were key to reentering home life.

Dick did not investigate rehabilitation facilities before his first heart attack. He was fortunate to have a bed at one of the best centers. At the same time, Larry, others, and I settled for uncertified facilities for therapy care due to ignorance and not performing interviews or walkthroughs.

Concerning story: The facility may hire an outside, subcontracted physical and occupational therapy company. Depending on the contract, the subcontractor will charge the facility or your insurance company by the hours each staff member works with you.

My first rehabilitation facility was not accredited. The subcontractor for PT and OT was the *second-worst* I experienced out of twelve facilities I went to. When they asked me to come out of the room for therapy, it was a demand, not a request. Beware of the contracted PT and OT if they are motivated by billable hours. These are hours that they can document for the rehabilitation facilities management and get paid.

Read the Joint Commission's Medicare nursing home care reports (https://www.medicare.gov/nursinghomecompare).

Reassuring story: When I was nearing the end of my stay at the CareAll facility, the last milestone for PT was walking up and down fourteen steps to the second floor with crutches. When using a cane or crutches, you need to put the weak foot down when stepping down a flight of stairs. The phrase I had to learn was "Down with the bad – up with the good." But during practice, I led with my good foot, and my legs gave out because my body weight shifted and the leg with the new implant buckled from the weight. Thanks to their training, the physical therapists walking with me held the gait belt and stopped me from tumbling down ten more steps.

I still had to reach the milestone of walking up and downstairs to be released from the facility. I was teamed up with a different therapist named Doreen, who heard about the fall. She went to the closet, took out some bright-colored tape, and placed it on my bad foot. The bad foot's visual impact constantly reminded me to go "down with the bad, up with the good."

Finally, I was discharged and used the tape for walking the steps at home for three more weeks. The two physical therapists prevented a life-threatening fall and then trained me with a clever technique — tape on my foot — to avoid falling after discharge. They may have saved my life.

Sean, a cancer survivor, who worked out at the YMCA, said, "Now that a pacemaker is in my chest, there specific motions that I should not do. The physical therapists reminded me that I should not reach above my head, so the wires and tubes implanted in my chest would not move or disconnect. They taught me how to get around those limitations. We practiced the levels and amount of time I could use various tools such as the treadmill and the stationary bike. I feel good that I can still come here and use these things. It makes me feel alive."

As Sean and I continued our conversation, it became apparent that he went to the same rehabilitation facility in Millbury mentioned above.

During your rehabilitation facility walkthrough, if there is a limited quality or quantity of tools to use in the physical and occupational therapy department, you should rate the facility poorly and be avoided. Check your insurance and understand how you are covered or your limitations on physical or occupational therapy. I list the suggested PT and OT equipment in Chapter Two.

The recreation department: www.recreationtherapy.org says that "recreational therapy, also known as therapeutic recreation, is a systematic process that [uses] recreation and other activity-based interventions to address the assessed needs of individuals with illnesses and/or disabling conditions, as well as psychological and physical health, recovery, and well-being."

Rosey, who was the head of the recreation at a MetroWest facility in Marlborough, Massachusetts, commented, "A good recreation department strives to help the men and women forget why they are at the facility. Whether they make crafts or listen to music, in their minds, they are people living ordinary, everyday lives."

A day in a rehabilitation facility usually has a pattern.

> 6 a.m. to 8 a.m. – wake up, bathroom, vitals, breakfast, and medicine by an RN
> 8 a.m. to 12 noon – PT or OT, meds, open time
> 12 noon to 1 p.m. – lunch
> 1 to 5 p.m. – meds, PT or OT, and open time

Physical and occupational therapy lasts typically one hour each unless you are at an acute rehabilitation facility. Your free time may be filled by showers, doctor/RN/CNA checkups, advocates, and family visits, but most days, you will have free time for at least four hours. You can walk the halls, read, watch TV, or work on a computer tablet, yet it is the period in the day in which self-pity, depression, recognition of pain, and thoughts of a poor outcome can become uppermost in your mind. All are mentally harmful and do not help with your recovery.

Why is therapeutic recreation significant? "Through the recreational activity, therapy recreation contributes to a healthier mind and body; makes life more satisfying and fun; and enables the [patient] to maintain a sense of wellness. Most importantly, TR empowers participants to enjoy life and reach their goals every day!" (Wikipedia)

I could not have worded its importance in a better way!

Ruth, a friend of Rosey, who worked in recreation for many years, is passionate about what recreation can do for the patient. "The recreation personnel and director must always greet any new patient who arrives at the facility, creating a sense of normalcy and comfort through the staff's friendly interaction and approach to the patient. Let the other departments know that recreation is available for short-term and permanent patient care."

Depending on your illness, the facility surroundings, atmosphere, and ecosystems contribute to a healthy mind and body. Make the best of your free time.

The patient's perspective: When you and your advocate interview the rehabilitation facilities, make sure there is a recreation department.

I spent four and a half months, during my first hip infection, at the Westborough facility. Only one person worked in the recreation department. The activities were "Guess the words, How many synonyms for a word, and Bingo." It was so bad that the director asked me to be the morning and evening facility announcer and assist with the word games; I was a patient. The correlation is obvious. No recreation during rehabilitation for the short- and long-term residents will be unsatisfactory for good health.

Concerns to look for: Recreation is an essential part of your interview checklist. Watch out for a rehabilitation facility with the following negative attributes:

- There is no recreation department.
- There is no calendar of events or activities.
- There are no tools to work with for recreational activities.
- The recreation department has staff but no departmental space.
- A subcontracted recreation staff is paid by billable hours.

Not all subcontracted recreation companies are bad. It would help if you asked whether the facility invested in certified staffing and resources to keep patients occupied. A subcontractor may insist that individuals participate; being pressured could spark depression and increase feelings of isolation. The participants in recreation should want to be there.

Ruth worked for a rehabilitation center with adequate tools and space for four years. Due to a reduced budget, the director had to cut corners in staff and routines. Corporate was negligent for not providing funding that would have delivered the facility's recreation objectives. The outsourced management gave orders to adjust the procedures for documentation and accreditation. Ruth stated, "For an extended period, the director highly suggested that her staff just visit one or two rooms on each wing and document a room visit. If the room was empty, the rule was to write in the activity document 'Patient not available.' As far as the facility was concerned, the boxes on the form had been checked for the state, Medicare/Medicaid, and Joint Commission visitation reports."

Uplifting experiences: As a resident of these facilities twelve times, I can tell you that benefits to the mind and body cannot be measured. It took at least six facilities for me to recognize recreation as necessary. Once I did, whether I was in the wheelchair or on crutches, I was at the recreation department for every activity that met my criteria.

During your walkthrough, look for:

- They write and print a daily newspaper to help residents learn about the organization and staff.
- They offer singing, crafts, puzzles, and other activities, including a library of books, magazines, and newspapers.
- They show old movies – for short- and long-term patients; movies bring back memories.

- They provide opportunities to play bingo games. This can have an uplifting effect. People with fewer cognitive skills can also play a version that has larger letters and numbers. Staff should be supportive and helpful to those who have difficulty following such games.

At CareAll, I created long-lasting friendships with people like Cat Johnson, who kept me in good spirits during the four times I was at the Millbury Massachusetts facility. We developed a strong friendship.

I met Steve and Paul during two of my stays at a facility outside Worcester, Massachusetts. Steve had a knee infection and Paul a hip infection, and both required skilled nursing for six weeks. This was their first stay at a post-acute rehabilitation facility, and they were both bored, complaining, and unhappy.

We struck up conversations. I insisted they both come with me to the recreation functions, and each of them agreed and went along with me. Both Steve and Paul became the most popular recreation patients in the facility. Steve commented to me before his discharge, "Recreation kept me busy, downplayed the pain, and cheered me up for weeks."

Should you stay longer than five days, recreation must be a vital consideration in a decision.

The conclusion: If there is no recreational department, you should rate the facility poorly and avoid it.

The Patient's Role – when the diagnosis is confirmed

The patient's role can range from submissive to controlling behavior. The following topics below are to suggest ways to be a better patient and, at the same time, know your rights. Defining your role is meant to let the medical professionals understand that you will participate in recovery and attempt to work with the professionals as a team member.

Due diligence is required: Wikipedia's definition of due diligence is, "The investigation or exercise of care that a reasonable business or person is expected to take before entering into any agreement or contract with another party, or an act with a certain standard of care. It can be a legal obligation, but the term will more commonly apply to voluntary investigations."

Let us take the keywords from the definition that define the expectations and intent of pre-surgical patients, advocates, and supporters:

Investigation – reasonable – expected – before entering -- an act – standard of care.

Those keywords define the obligation of any individual to be an activist and advocate for themselves. If you have the time, ability, and wherewithal, you must act for the benefit of a positive outcome from your illness and investigate. Be aware that many medical professionals and facilities will not receive your questions with open arms. If there is resistance to your due diligence, it should raise a red flag about their business, personalities, and behaviors.

Remember the cardiac patient, Dick Maggio, who went to Beth Israel Hospital for surgery on his heart? Dick had to have two operations before his final discharge. He knew nothing about the hospital's physical therapy, and he knew nothing about the quality of a rehabilitation facility before being admitted the first time. Dick told me, "I knew squat about the nurses and what they do." Yet, Dick was delighted with the acute-care facility because of the quality of care he received and his recovery results.

Had Dick performed due diligence on the Braintree facility, using the Joint Commission's Quality Reports and *Medicare.gov/nursinghomecompare*, he would have found that his facility had accreditation for "Nursing Care" and "Acute Care," which were what Dick needed.

Tools are available to perform due diligence on hospitals, rehabilitation facilities, surgeons, and staff positions. Other than the need for a spontaneous operation beyond your control, the choice is yours.

Spontaneous need for an operation: The day after I was told that I needed a double revision, I knew, from speaking with surgeons and infectious disease professionals, that I had no choice but to have the operations. If I refused, sepsis could poison the blood, and I would die. So, I listed the hospitals I would investigate and acquired a list of rehabilitation facilities from each hospital's social services representative.

I wasted no time and started to list questions for the surgeons and recruited Pat B. as my note-taking advocate. Within a week, we visited three hospitals and three surgeons. Then I started to interview the rehabilitation facilities on my list.

The pain in the right hip increased so much by the second rehab facility that I asked a good friend, Mike Rizzo, to drive me to the remaining rehab facilities. Before getting out of the car, my pain was 7 and 8 on the medical pain level linear scale. It was just too much pain. I asked Mike to take me to the Newton hospital, which I had visited three days before. We walked into the emergence room, and I notified the emergency room nurses and doctors that Dr. William Henderson, the orthopedic surgeon, was my doctor. I was now linked to Dr. Henderson, whom I chose due to previous interviews. The X-ray had shown that the stem of the first implant on the right hip had become loose. The stem was moving and touching the infected areas inside the hip. I described the pain as feeling like someone made an incision with a dull knife, 8 inches long, and stuck a finger into my body, and was wiggling the finger.

Whether it is cancer, infections, or a heart attack, the spontaneous need for hospitalization would interfere with finishing the interview process. Still, while you are in the hospital, your advocate will have a minimum of three days to interview and decide on the best rehabilitation facility for your care. Without help in completing due diligence, you are at the mercy of the social service associate at the hospital. They will provide a physical rehabilitation facility list that you would have to throw darts at to make a choice; you are guessing.

It was fortunate that I had had seven other operations and learned the hard way to carry out investigations. Should you have the time, do *not* do what I did, that is, nothing. In the first four operations, I trusted the people who had recommended the surgeons.

After that, the hospital social workers sent me to a rehab facility of their choice, and it was a hellhole. The result was an infection, pain, and disability. Should there be enough time to do the work, you can make a confident decision.

Commitment and the advocate's value: When you are diagnosed with an illness, a commitment must be made. There should be a total agreement among the hospital, surgeon, and the medical team whether you require stents for the arteries or urine track, open-heart surgery, orthopedic work, or any other procedures that are intrusive to your body. Physical and mental commitment should be your primary focus.

You must get the reports from every consultation. In addition, request orders from various departments for x-rays, MRIs, and CT scans. Even at the best hospitals, orders from the surgeons can contain inaccurate statements in the report or show the wrong pictures.

During a particularly important part of the revision process, X-rays were ordered for me. Don Hanssen, my advocate, escorted me to the radiology department, which he had done many times before. At this visit, I asked the attendant to read what parts of the body images would be taken. Much to our surprise, the orders sent from the orthopedic staff were for the wrong body parts. Don knew it, and so did I. The fact is, this happens, so be preemptive. The benefit of bringing an advocate is the verification of the mistake, a second opinion, and helping to restore confidence and commitment.

You can ask: *why, what for, and what the severe after-effects are,* but it is necessary to know the following steps of the procedure. Ask your advocate to be at the meeting as a stenographer and observer. Write down all stages of the process and continue to research the information about what is being done.

The commitment to the process must be a "let's get it done" attitude. Let the radiologist do their job and cooperate entirely with all pre-surgical personal questions, blood tests, swab tests, diets, and pre-surgical medicines. Follow doctors' requests for pre-operation procedures at home. These must be done and are just as important as the surgery.

An essential "must-do" is bathing with soap or antiseptic that the hospital prescribes to sanitize the body before the operation(s). The cleaning is usually done every day for a specified duration; three to five days is standard. If you have a partner or advocate at your residence, ask them to wash where you cannot reach.

If you have no advocate, organizations like the Visiting Nurses or Visiting Angels can help you sterilize your body.

Commitment is a mental attitude that motivates you to do whatever it takes for a favorable outcome.

Impatience and anxiety: You enter a different world when it's necessary to interact with the medical field, especially in a specialized environment. At some point during the experience, impatience will take over. Your impatience and anxiety may push your advocate, partner, family, and friends into an indifferent attitude. This is the support you cannot allow to escape.

Potentially, the mind will race, imaging negative outcomes that are inaccurate and cause fear. This behavior will work against the talent of your medical professionals.

Behavior examples to stay away from:

- Calling the surgeon too often.
- Calling the surgeon's physician assistant and nurse practitioner too often.
- Making appointments for reasons that do not exist, merely to feel better and ask questions that were already answered or irrelevant.
- Making an appointment or calling your primary doctor to reinforce whether you are doing the right things.
- Making the advocate, friends, and family upset by asking unnecessary questions and creating circumstances that do not exist.

These are samples of impatience, anxiety, and lack of confidence. This behavior will upset the individual roles of the people you asked to help and those you need for the process. If this anxiety becomes acute, people will begin to turn away.

Anxiety can become acute. Your body may start to shake, and depression or panic attacks could set in. This may advance the illness and inflame the problem.

Impatience and anxiety can reach a climax while you are waiting for the call of life or death. Sean, the member at my gym, was at the end of cancer and explained to me the need to control yourself. He said, "Bill, the waiting is like everything is in neutral. In the cancer environment, it is called a brain stop. You shut down activities for the future and live in the past or the present; you watch too much television."

It was as if Sean knew exactly what I went through, waiting to know if the hip infections were gone. I got my affairs in order, stopped all plans, and arranged for my son to be notified as carefully as possible. Sean and I won our battles. We were humbled and resumed our lives.

The takeaway from the story is to do what it takes to reduce impatience and anxiety. Set a routine: Walk, run, go to the gym, or do your favorite activity. While raising my son Billy, I would tell him to face his fears, and he did. Now it was my time to set an example.

Know your medication: Not knowing precisely every pill or liquid medication will disable or kill you. You must know every pill, liquid, and hypodermic your doctor has prescribed by name and sight. You must write down your usual medication, antibiotics, and pain medication.

The complete list of medicines you take is indispensable and must always be known. These examples of botched information are valid instances of errors that were life-threatening. I separated the factual accounts into two areas: the primary doctor and the hospital.

The professional's misinformation: The report of all the medicines you take, including quantity, must be verified by you and your primary doctor, your specialty doctor's group, the advocate, and your family.

This is an example of database confusion.

The correct medicines prescribed were:

- Bupropion — 2 pills, twice a day
- Gabapentin for neuropathy — 3 pills in the morning; 2 pills in the afternoon; 1 pill before bed; a total of 7/day
- Sulfamethoxazole to suppress infection — 1 pill, twice a day

The report from my primary's system:

- Bupropion — 1 pill, twice a day
- Gabapentin for neuropathy — 2 capsules every 3 hours and 1 before bed for a total of 7/day
- Sulfamethoxazole to suppress infection — 1 pill, twice a day

The report of my medicine from the hospital and rehabilitation facility's computer system was:

- Bupropion — 1 pill, once a day
- Gabapentin for neuropathy — 4 400 mg capsules, once a day

- Sulfamethoxazole to suppress infection – 1 pill, twice a day

We are fortunate that the medical systems databases are integrated. As of this date, your primary's HMO or previous specialty physician can share information, such as previous visits, diagnosis, and medicines.

Should you go to another HMO or doctor for your operation, normally the primary's HMO data cannot be shared unless you give them the authority to do so. In my case, the work to correct the reports was mine. I met with all the infectious disease medicine assistants, and we entered the correct data. I urge you to keep checking reports for errors.

Changes in medication prescribed over time and reported between departments may be outdated. It is a fact that the potential for error is when different medical assistances enter the data over time. I allowed the two HMOs to share the data and reports of all my meds, and the data was still inaccurate. In addition to the problem, the false data was transferred to the rehabilitation facility. During the consultations before my operation, I recognized the issue and then worked with each medical professional to have the correct time, number, brand, and quantity of meds for everyone.

Your responsibility is to correct this confusion as time goes by. The easiest way to manage the issue is to double-check that the doctor's reports are correct in every meeting with the primary, surgeons, nurse practitioners, rehab facilities, and home care attendants. It is your responsibility to make multiple copies of your meds and put them in familiar places such as a designated drawer, backpack, purse, luggage, and with your advocates. You should show the copy to all medical professionals during any consultation.

Confront institutional arrogance: During one of my visits as a volunteer at a rehabilitation facility, a patient confided in me how he became his advocate. Larry from Lowell, Massachusetts, knew his medicine by its name, pill color, shape, and quantity.

Larry had just been transferred from a first rehabilitation facility outside Lowell (a one-star rehab) to a four-star facility outside Worcester, where I befriended him. Larry told me what happened to him at his first facility, "Bill, it was time for night pills before I went to bed. The floor nurse brought my pills in a plastic container. I said to the nurse, "Sorry, these are not my meds, so go back and get the right pills!" The nurse insisted that they were the correct medicines. This disagreement went on for 15 minutes.

"I ordered her to get the head night nurse immediately. The head nurse insisted the floor nurse was correct. At this point, I raised my voice and said, "I demand to see the director of nursing," Both left the room, with an attitude of superiority. I thought they were calling the director; 20 minutes later, the two returned. In the head nurse's hand was a plastic container with pills of the correct color, shape, and quantity! They were the right meds! Bill, one must be their own advocate. Both nurses apologized to me for their attitude and having the wrong meds. Someone should write a book on all this!"

Here is a perfect example of how the professional and the patient clash. Larry was a self-advocate and held his ground. The nurses refused to listen, but it ended well because Larry knew his medications. Larry's comment reinforced my desire to write this book.

In Doctor Edward Hoffer's book, *Prescription for Bankruptcy*, he writes, the medical professionals are overburdened, especially in the ICU. For example, a patient at the Good Samaritan in Brockton, Massachusetts, was severely allergic to a particular drug. This was noted in the record, and even though both the pharmacists dispensing the drug and the nurse administrating it got computer "pop-ups" stating the allergy, they gave him the drug. Fortunately, the patient recovered, but only after being rushed to the ICU.

A warning pop-up on the computer screen may occur dozens or even hundreds of times a day. However, after a while, it is easy to tune these out as false alarms.

Patients! Always know your meds and have the correct list with you!

Symptoms and pain: The definition of symptoms and pain can be synonymous. When a symptom starts to emerge, pain may happen at the same time. "Many illnesses or disorders, such as flu, fibromyalgia, irritable bowel syndrome (IBS), and reproductive issues, can cause pain. Some people experience other symptoms with pain. These can include nausea, dizziness, fatigue, loss of appetite, irritability, depression, and anger." (Healthline.com)

Symptoms and pain (S&P) may vary widely depending on the injury, operation, or illness. Whether it is pancreatic cancer, colitis, bone-on-bone joints, symptoms can signify substantial illness and more pain. After surgery, orthopedic symptoms of concern are redness around the incision, hotness to the touch, pus coming from the incision, and bubbles filled with pus.

Those symptoms were from my first infection on the left hip, which the doctors suppressed by prescribing Sulfamethoxazole-trimethoprim; the signs and pain disappeared. Months later, after surgery, the right hip became infected, and I had no symptoms until six months later; then, there was just nagging pain. Pain became the symptom. The antibiotic could not suppress two severely infected hips, so the pain, redness, and burning heat were symptoms of a much more complex problem than before.

If possible, your role is to get three opinions from specialty doctors, depending on the symptoms or pain. Should spontaneous symptoms and pain begin, call 911 or an emergency medical technician (EMT) as quickly as possible. When S&P starts, engage a medical professional.

> **The reality of symptoms and pain:** My S&P was straightforward. Each symptom indicated an infection. Signs of the first infection started; I engaged an infectious disease doctor, and he suppressed the pain. I did not want

a surgical reversal, so taking antibiotics for the rest of my life was fine with me, but when the second infection's symptoms and pain started with the second implant, I had no choice but surgery.

I had a roommate, Langley, at a rehab during my fight to eliminate infections. Langley had a stroke in New Hampshire, which resulted in symptoms, but he ignored them for a short time until his arm went limp, his speech became slurred, and there was numbing in his face. Unfortunately, Langley suffered a worse condition by not calling for help sooner.

My outcome was that I survived after suffering pain at Level 9 on the pain scale and acted after some time went by. Langley's outcome was lengthy physical and occupational therapy; he came back 70%. We had symptoms, but we did not engage medical professionals as quickly as possible, so we suffered the consequences.

The common denominator for both of us was that we did not do the right things at the right time. As a result, Langley may have had minor damage to his body. I could have eliminated the first infection and possibly have gone to another surgeon for the second hip, saving me a year of additional operations and pain.

Langley and I failed to understand and act upon our role as patients. As a result, we ignored symptoms and will suffer for life.

Learn and use the pain level scale: Pain must be qualified by the people suffering from it. A book called *The Patient's Perspective* says, "I think a scale of 1 to 10 is a poor tool for assessing chronic conditions whose symptoms are variable."

Pain can be variable or changeable. The definition of variable as an adjective:

"not consistent or having a fixed pattern; liable to change, able to be changed or adapted."

As a noun:
an element, feature, or factor that is liable to vary or change.
"There are too many variables involved to make any meaningful predictions." (ProOxford dictionary)

The keywords are "liable to change" and "liable to vary or change." Once the pain begins, you need to set a baseline. Should the pain spike or rotate, the pain is still there, which means a baseline before the spike or rotation can be set. When enduring an *intense* pain spike or rotation of pain, you can set a higher level. Then, you can communicate the accuracy of the two pain levels correctly to the doctors.

The 1 to 10 pain scale pertains to any pain for any medical condition of the body. Each symptom and illness have relative feelings of pain and discomfort. Pain levels have a baseline, midpoint, acute, and then chronic level. For example, if a patient has stomach cancer, it may first feel like stomachache, which can be used as a baseline of 1 to 3; when the burning starts, it is at a different level of 4 to 6. When the pain feels like a knife in your body, you can communicate the pain level to the doctors as 8 or 9.

During my battle with hip infections, sometimes there would be no pain, especially when I was sitting down. But when I became more active or had to travel, the pain became unbearable. The pain level scale is a suitable method for self-analyzing to communicate correctly with the medical professional.

You can learn more at https://www.healthline.com/health/pain-scale. They do an excellent job of describing levels of pain.

Levels of pain may begin in the hip, knee, and leg, with heat inside the affected area (levels 1 to 3); you are functional. Sometime later, the same region may have a dull, uncomfortable, and constant pain (levels 3 to 5). Then sometime later, the infected area and bone feel a sharp, sporadic pain like a knife is inside, and you only want to sit and cannot sleep (levels five to7). Finally, the infection can escalate to a level you want to scream, cry, and cannot walk without help (levels 7 to 9).

After-surgery pain scale: From your own experience, you can learn your pain level for an illness. The post-operative professionals and surgeons will continue to ask about your pain level. Know it and be truthful.

The post-operation pain level scale is significant for the PT and OT departments. Your pain level statement will let them know what you can work with at a baseline level. As was stated earlier, PT and OT can dictate your discharge. It is recommended not to play any pain level games with them.

You will be pleasantly surprised to find that therapy works, and pain levels decrease when you are honest.

If the surgeons and rehabilitation professionals have determined that your residence is safe for your recovery, they will suggest home care and outsourced physical therapy. Pain levels will be used when you are having home care nursing and physical therapy. The pain scale system will apply, but it should be at the lower range if the operation went well enough for you to have home care. Again, be truthful.

Beware that pain may not be an indicator of a problem: Pain is relevant to each patient. Kim O'Brien considered her pain to be mild and rated it a 2. The last surgeon she went to listened to her symptoms, disregarded her interpretation of the pain level, and ordered further tests. It was the last test, a CT scan, that led to diagnosing the correct problem. The severity of the symptoms was alarming to the specialist – not the patient's interpretation of the pain levels.

Kim's symptoms: dizzy spells, tingling/numbness in arms, legs, and face. Very mild pain in the neck area, muscle tightness, and occasional mild nerve pain.

Eventually, her symptoms, which were not painful, became acute, and Kim collapsed to the floor in front of a class. It was a symptom that pushed the search for another surgical opinion.

She said, "One day, I was at work, and both my legs went completely numb. I felt like I could barely walk right. I decided that was it. I was headed to the last neurosurgeon on my list. I made the appointment and went in the next week." Kim O'Brien was a self-advocate.

She went for multiple recommendations and did not stop at just one or two opinions. Instead, she took her records with her, researched each surgeon's background, found the real problem through additional tests, and made the correct decision.

The takeaway from this section is that pain was not an indicator; it was the symptoms. The process for addressing the symptoms is just the same as a severe pain illness. You need to follow the multiple-opinion process of the investigation.

Hope — Fight — Live are three words that make up "the patient's role"!

CHAPTER TWO

INPATIENT REHABILITATION FACILITY (IRF) OR SKILLED NURSING FACILITY (SNF)

A**cute and Skilled Nursing Facilities:** Acute (IRF) and Skilled Nursing Facilities, also known as post-acute care, are defined by Bellavistahealth.com as an "inpatient rehabilitation facility which offers acute care for those who need a higher level of rehabilitation following traumatic injuries and surgeries such as amputations. On the other hand, skilled nursing facilities provide post-acute rehabilitation, which is similar but less intensive than the therapies provided at an IRF."

I have interviewed a fair number of (Acute) Inpatient Rehabilitation Facilities (IRFs), but I resided in Skilled Nursing Facilities (SNFs). You should be comforted that IRFs are qualified to handle challenging cases. The hospital and the surgeons will suggest the type of facility you should be admitted to. **My goal is to for you to know the difference.**

Acute rehabilitation: The IRF will typically be a much larger rehabilitation facility than an SNF. Along with the facility's size, the resources available to you are more diverse than the SNF. For example, the physical therapy area will use equipment that is specific to your injury. During my visits to the physical therapy area, I saw intensive tools such as walking-assist belt systems to keep patients from falling. In addition, there was a half-car for patients to learn the correct way of entering and exiting a car. The staff is trained in and familiar with acute rehabilitation techniques for patients afflicted with a stroke, quadruple heart bypass, debilitating diseases, and severe trauma. Acute care also provides occupational and speech therapy. One of the differentiators of the IRF (acute care) is that the schedules are predetermined and consist of doctors, nurses, PTs, and OTs for specific hours in the day. The doctors are one-on-one for mandatory daily consultations.

Skilled Nursing Facility (sub-acute; post-acute care): "In an acute rehabilitation program, patients receive physical, occupational, and speech therapy as needed. Skilled Nursing Facility/Post-Acute rehabilitation is less intense than acute rehabilitation. Patients in a subacute facility generally only receive one or two hours of therapy per day, and it is a combination of physical, occupational, and speech therapy. At a SNF (post-acute facility), the hours of therapy are random and scheduled that day. The therapy department informs you of your schedule in the morning.

You see the attending physician at admission, once during your stay, and at discharge." (Gwinnett Medical Center)

The new term for subacute rehabilitation is post-acute care. The terms post-acute care and post-acute rehabilitation will be used as you read on. The new term may not be found in other articles or "Googling," but they have the same meaning.

I met with Dan D., director of admissions at an acute-care facility in Braintree, Massachusetts. His explanation of the quality of care at his facility was, "In this type of care facility, we receive patients who have illnesses that are intense and life-threatening, such as heart attack and strokes. When a patient is admitted to our facility and has gone through the admitting process and room assignment, there is intense care every day. For example, the doctor who has the patient meets one on one every day. The rehabilitation will run three hours a day or potentially two three-hour sessions a day."

The need for an inpatient rehabilitation facility came into my family's lives. John, my brother, was driving home to Skaneateles, New York when his SUV was slammed on the side by a V-shaped plow driven by a drunk driver. John was only bruised and had neck pain.

As time went by, he started to experience more internal complications from the accident. At one point, he fell and broke his hip. John's primary physician, affiliated with a Syracuse hospital, admitted him to a post-acute care facility. The hospital and the primary treated him for the hip and superficial damage.

As time passed, it became evident that his health was in decline. At that time, Jane, John's daughter, and Julia, his wife, with the help of a sister in Atlanta and her nurse practitioner friend, Lisa H., teamed together and set up plans for visiting and interviewing acute and subacute hospitals in the area.

John's acute issues had to be addressed, so they crossed off the use of skilled nursing facilities. Instead, they decided on visiting two acute (IRF) rehabilitation facilities. The family became dissatisfied with the primary doctor's choice of care and took it upon themselves to create a list of criteria and resources to visit to interview different doctors and facilities. They devised a list and crossed off one IRF because of deficiencies in the physical therapy department, the rooms, poor food service, and the orderly dining area.

I was highly impressed with the excellent work they did. The family became the advocates for a man who could not do it himself. The family and friends used many of the decision criteria you will read about below.

Searching for an Inpatient Rehabilitation Facility (IRF)

Suppose you know the severity of your operation, trauma, or disease in advance. In that case, you have the advantage of choosing a facility by using the methods described in the following sections. Of course, should you become ill quickly, chances are you will not have the advantage of deciding on the facility you will go to, but that does not mean you should not explore acute and subacute facilities are in your area.

Jane and Julia realized that the hospital's care, referred by John's primary care doctor, was unsatisfactory and not equipped with appropriate resources. They visited two other IRF's and decided on the best one. They discarded John's current hospital and the primary doctor's services for the acute care facility's talent and experience. This facility discovered that John was bleeding in the brain, which had to be addressed and cognitive tests implemented.

Rich, who had a quadruple bypass operation, was sent to an IRF south of Boston when he had his first heart event. Since the event occurred so fast, the choice was not his to make. A second operation was planned, and Rich had time to investigate other IRF organizations. Yet, Rich was pleased with the first IRF experience; he returned to South Boston.

The following sections apply to either the IRF or the SNF. It is the severity of the illness that determines the level of care. If you know the diagnosis early, the best step you can take is to ask the specialty doctor what they recommend.

Searching for a Skilled Nursing Rehabilitation Facility

I met Steve during one of my stays at a rehabilitation facility. Steve told me that the hospital recommended the rehabilitation facility he would go to since he did not know how to choose one. During his stay at that rehabilitation facility, his wound was left open for two days. Worrying about infection, Steve took phone pictures of the open thigh, forwarded the images to his surgeon, and with a phone call,

Steve was sent to an accredited rehabilitation facility – the facility where I stayed. The surgeons closed the open wound, increased antibiotics, and raised the probability of a better recovery.

Steve admitted that he had not done his due diligence on a rehabilitation facility before the operation. He and I checked the rehab facilities recommended by a hospital social services person from the Medicare report. Steve's first rehab was on the list, but it only had one star and unacceptable reports.

Methods of searching for the rehabilitation facility: I was a patient at twelve rehabilitation and long-term care facilities. In my case, it was a foregone conclusion that I would need skilled care**. Therefore, this chapter is focused on addressing the need for a physical rehabilitation facility.**

The definition of a physical rehabilitation facility is "medicine and rehabilitation (PM&R). Also known as physiatry or rehabilitation medicine, it aims to enhance and restore functional ability and quality of life to those with physical impairments or disabilities affecting the brain, spinal cord, nerves, bones, joints, ligaments, muscles, and tendons." (Wikipedia)

Note: Researching the physical rehabilitation and long-term care facility is like the "Searching for a Hospital" section of this book.

Talking and listening: Talking to individuals and family members you know and trust. You may narrow down the three physical rehabs to visit with advice from those people. The concern you should have with this method is whether the care facility "is right for me and my illness." By investigating a minimum of three facilities, you will know which one has the tools, skilled professionals, and a healthy environment for your return to a good quality of life.

A hospital's social and services representative: The healthcare nurse will have a list of inpatient rehab facilities within a preset distance from the hospital. Each of the facilities is rated by Medicare stars. The more significant amount of stars, the better. Contact the social services manager and acquire that list *before*_the operation. You will now have a resource to decide on the three rehabs to visit. For additional options, I suggest asking for the list of those that are farther from the hospital and are still acceptable to you, your family, your advocate, and your insurance.

The internet and cloud technology: Technology are tools to investigate rehabilitation facilities. It would help if you Googled the rehab care and long-term care websites within a geographic area that you and your advocate targeted. You may have to be transported back and forth to the hospital for a checkup or an emergency, so the hospital's distance should assist in narrowing the search. If you choose within 25 miles, search it; if you decide within 50 miles, explore it.

My best experience was 40 miles outside of Boston in Millbury, MA.

Concerns with an internet search: When using the internet and clicking on websites, they typically portray the organization as having the best-skilled nurses, an enjoyable environment, post-hospital care, and recovery. You will find that the sites represent themselves as Tier One organizations. Each search of the facilities will put a happy face on a tough decision in your life. Use the internet only as a research source; for example, one rehab facility had more to offer, such as recreation, hairdressing, and free transportation. Once you have qualified a facility on paper, the onsite visit is your next step.

Medicare.gov/nursinghomecompare: Nursing Home Compare allows you to find and compare nursing homes certified by Medicare and Medicaid. This website contains the quality of resident care and staffing information for more than 15,000 nursing homes worldwide. Nursing homes provide skilled care to people who cannot be cared for at home and need 24-hour nursing care. Most of these facilities include skilled nursing and post-acute care for rehabilitation.

Please note that the description "nursing home" also pertains to post-acute care/skilled nursing rehabilitation facilities.

"Skilled care includes skilled nursing or rehabilitation services to manage, observe, or assess a resident's care. Examples of skilled care include occupational therapy, wound care, intravenous (IV) therapies, and physical therapy." (www.cms.gov)

The information on Nursing Home Compare can help you learn:

- How nursing homes have performed in health and fire safety inspections.
- How the nursing home is staffed with nurses and other healthcare providers.
- How well nursing homes care for their residents.
- Nursing homes that have had issues related to preventing abuse.
- Nursing homes with significant issues maintaining compliance to protect resident health and safety and are part of the Special Focus Facility Program.

An actual comparison of two Massachusetts Post-Acute Care/SNF facilities: Below is a comparison of two skilled nursing facilities in Massachusetts. I have used two ZIP codes: 01581 and 01527. The ZIP codes correspond to the facilities.

These rehabilitation facilities are two of which I was a resident. ZIP code: 01581 was one of my first rehabilitation facilities; I resided there for four and a half months. ZIP code: 01527 is the rehabilitation facility I stayed at four separate times due to my infected hips. At my request, I returned to 01527 for a total of 225 days.

The number of health inspection citations is essential to determine an acceptable choice. These charts, provided by medicare.gov/compare, compare many topics, statistics, and qualifications of a facility.

How do we use the Medicare.gov website: The following should help you drill down into the relevant data you require for rehabilitation facilities and nursing homes. Note: you can compare more than two facilities at once.

1. *Go to medicare.gov/nursinghomecompare.*
2. *Click on "Nursing homes including rehab facilities.*
3. *Type in the area you would like to investigate (you can choose near the hospital or near your advocate and your home. Anywhere you feel the facility you want is located – in this case, zip code 01581/Westborough)*
4. *There are five tabs you can choose from to search/filter criteria you decide to focus on. Distance in miles: Overall rates (star ratings); Other ratings (star rating by categories – Health inspection, staffing, and quality of care); several beds; more filters.*
5. *The system will provide many facilities to choose from. Click on the first facility you would like to compare. In this case the Westboro facility. Then, click the "compare" tab.*
6. *Scroll down till you find the second facility you would like to compare. In this case, zip code: 01527/Millbury. Then, click on the "compare" tab.*
7. *In the upper right-hand corner, click compare.*
8. *The first screen provides relevant data about each facility. Then, scrolling down, you will find data/information*

categories to investigate (health inspection, staffing, quality of resident care, fire safety, and penalties).

9. *The chart below contains data from "overall rating and quality of resident care.*

Nursing and Rehabilitation Facility	Star rating	Health inspection # of citations in 2019	Pneumonia prevention % of short-stay needing and getting the flu shot	Flu prevention: % of short-stay needing and got a vaccine to prevent flu	% of a successful return to home and community for an SNF	% number of residents at or above-expected ability to move around at discharge.	
ZIP code: 01527	★★★★	9	99	99.1	66.4	40.6	
ZIP code: 01581	★	16	17%	41	28	54.8	
National Average		8.2	76.6	0*	50.1	48.5	

**Scores above 0 mean that the self-care score has improved, and scores below 0 mean that the self-care score has worsened.*

Breakfast for ZIP code: 01581-rehabilitation facility – degrading recovery.

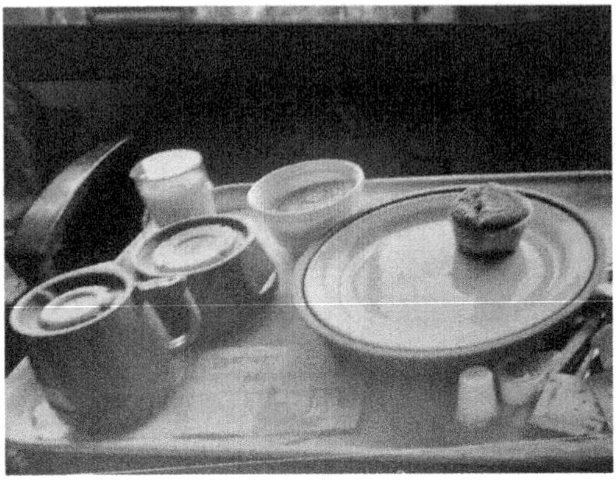

From William R. Butler's personal photo vault

Breakfast for ZIP code: 01527 rehabilitation facility – uplifting for a good recovery.

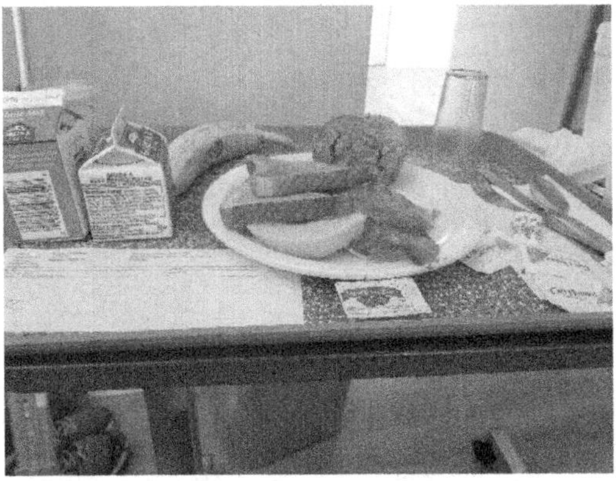

From William R. Butler's personal photo vault

The more you study the resources and information available to you, the more variables you will discover a facility provides. It is up to you, your advocate, and your doctor to decide what categories and data are essential for your care.

The Joint Commission on Health Organization: The Joint Commission website and search engines are also suitable for gathering relevant reports for selecting a facility. The Joint Commission website will guide you to other websites that rate rehabilitation facilities in detail. You will have access to doctors and the HMOs with which they are affiliated. You will be able to view and print the reports that pertain to your condition and whether that health organization has the "Gold Seal."

This is an example of researching information: Google "Joint Commission" – click "Quality Care" – Search – Rehabilitation Center in Braintree, Massachusetts – Report: nursing care is accredited – detail." The quality reports also date the "last onsite survey date." For example, the Braintree Center's last date was 2019. In Marlborough, Massachusetts, the rehabilitation facility submitted its last survey in 2017. Therefore, the Marlborough facility survey is out of date.

The importance of onsite visits and interviews

Once the off-site research has been done, and chosen three rehabilitation and nursing care facilities, call the admissions director of each facility. Make an appointment and gather all the web reports, plus information from friends and your advocate. List questions to ask and departments you would like to see.

Your advocate should go with you on the visits. The advocate will document the topics discussed with the admissions director. During the onsite rehabilitation visit, the advocate should take notes of all the departments you visit. If the director allows it, take pictures, but due to HIPAA and the patients' privacy, pictures may not be allowed; what you see may have to be written down.

The onsite visit will open your eyes to the facility's reality and nursing experience. It allows you to use your senses to assist in the decisions you are about to make.

Questions to ask: After making the appointments, write up a list of relevant questions to take with you. My suggestion is to use your time efficiently and not list or ask questions about anything can see clearly.

A sample of questions:

- How can we reserve a bed?
- How many registered nurses (RNs) are on the floor each shift?
- How are many certified nursing assistants (CNAs) are on the floor each shift?
- What is the ratio of RNs and CNAs to patients on the floor?
- How do the nurses and/or management check to see if meds are delivered on time?
- Which practices are Joint Commission Gold Seal-certified?

- Could I see a food service menu and/or an alternative menu?
- Could I see a real meal?
- Could we visit the physical and occupational therapy departments?
- Could we visit the recreational department?
- Could we have a recreational department calendar of events for the month?

The advocates for my brother, John, listed additional questions and observations:

- Do they have a kitchen and dining area?
- Do they have private rooms, and how many?
- How do they schedule physical therapy appointments? Do the patients wait in lines?
- If the patient misses a scheduled appointment (due to showering or other required activity), can they reschedule for that day?
- What is the neighborhood like? Does it have safe parking? What does the parking cost?
- Can the patient have access to an air mattress bed to reduce bedsores?
- Is the bathroom shared with another patient or another room?

You can discuss admission and insurance questions before or after the walk-through. It would be best if you were insured. Go home, decide on the facility you rate as number 1, and rank the other two.

Once the facility looks like it could be your choice and the admission and insurance discussions are over, let the admissions director know how much you want to recover in his or her facility. *Ask how you can be assured a bed.*_The standard reply to this question is, "We can provide a bed if one is available at the time you are discharged from the hospital." Although that is the standard answer, follow up with a call to the director of admissions before the operation; reiterate your desire for a bed.

When I finally selected a facility, I called the director with my operation's date and added two or three days. This provides the estimated date that insurance is accepted for rehab after an operation. A few days before the operation, make another call to let the director know that the operation is a "go" and confirm the date. Your sincerity and relationship with the admissions director could make the difference between no bed and confirmation of availability. Be pleasant and not dictatorial or demanding. Remember that this is the manager who can help you with current and future surgeries.

> **Visit the physical and occupational therapy departments:** The process and descriptions that follow are based on a professional team with adequate equipment to do the job. Aspects of departments you should be cautious of will be in later stories.

During the first day of physical therapy meetings, you will be introduced to the staff and the director. At these meetings, you should have a two-way conversation about your goals and what they want to see in your abilities at discharge.

First, the therapist will work with you on the milestones to achieve the goals you all agree to. That information will be logged into a laptop or tablet for accurate information to measure your success and achieve your milestones. The therapist will ask you to perform several activities to set your performance baseline, which your milestones will be measured against. As challenging and painful as it is, you will want a baseline to experience positive reinforcement as you improve.

During your visit, confirm the routine described above. If that is missing, you should downgrade the department.

I will list pieces of equipment, practice areas, and comfortable areas to look for. Each one will be used by the physical and occupational therapist, depending upon your goals. During your visits, you will benefit from seeing firsthand the facility's capabilities and discussing the tools that should be used, based on the type of surgery you will be having.

(Physical therapy equipment is based on suggestions from the American Physical Therapy Association and the author.)

- Treatment tables: hard, not covered, wooden bed-size slab; high-low adjustable mat table; bed-size with pillows and blankets.
- Stationary bike with backward- and forward-resistance handgrips and petals.

- Window-sized rubber background net, used for rebounding pitching with different weight balls thrown and caught by you.
- Multilevel, adjustable stairs with railings; adjustable exercise stairs without railings
- Wall mirrors
- Tables for discussions, paperwork, and home eating practice
- Mobilization belts for different parts of the body
- Gait belts
- Parallel bars
- Real single bed and recliner chair
- Lift equipment for relearning how to stand
- Weights and resistant pulleys
- Medicine balls
- Playing cards

Occupational therapy home practice areas –

Kitchen:

- Sink with sponges, glass holders, and hand towels
- Cabinets with cups, dishes, bowls, and pans
- Drawers with utensils, knives, strainers, and oven gloves
- Cooking tools, toaster, microwave, cutting plates
- Refrigerator stocked with food and condiments for cooking
- Cupboards contain cooking materials such as flour, sugar, spices, and oils

- Stove
- Coffeemaker

Bathroom:

- Full-size bathtub with grab bars
- Toilet with support bars on the wall
- Sink for brushing teeth, shaving, and combing hair
- Bathtub containing transfer seat with adjustable chair
- Tub-mount swivels
- Sliding bath transfer bench
- Towels, fake razor, plastic-wrapped toothbrush

Everyday strengthening activity:

- Tool to measure distances you can walk with or without a walker, crutches, or cane
- Stretching belts for leg and arm strengthening

Coordination tools:

- Games for practicing dexterity, speed, and cognitive recognition
- Medical supplies: stethoscope, blood pressure cuff, tape measures, thermometers, defibrillator, and standard safety kits

Advanced tools:

- Indoor pool
- Lifting device for entering and exiting the pool and treadmill
- Simulated car for learning the correct way to enter and exit

The facility may hire a contracted physical therapy company with a good portion of the items mentioned above. Remember that the contracted physical and occupational therapists are motivated by billable hours; they document the facility, insurance, and state. The state uses these statistics for inspection and evaluation before deciding on accreditation.

You should view and understand the diversity of the rehabilitation tools and equipment investment in the facility to benefit your recovery. The tools you will use depend on prescriptions from the surgeon and the rehabilitation facility's doctor's orders; if a department is ill-equipped, take that organization off your list.

My preference is that the facility owns and is responsible for physical and occupational therapy. If they are owned by an organization focused on your recovery, they are the people you can point to if you need help or have a complaint.

Visit the recreation and food service departments:

Recreation: *A caring and well-funded facility should use these:*

- Calendar of recreational events
- Several trained recreational professionals
- Rooms strictly used for recreation
- Computers for the recreation staff
- Music groups, choirs, piano player, and facility planned events
- Clergy visits
- Games and effort activities:

- Bingo — one for the cognitive wing and one for the memory wing
- Puzzles, coloring, crossword puzzles, playing cards
- Music and pictures from past generations
- Charades, word games
- Crafts
- Dancing and sing-alongs

When you participate in recreational functions, you benefit by meeting others, improve cognitive awareness, reinforce retention, and encourage good humor, all of which improve recovery and wellness and avoid depression and loneliness.

Rosey, a member of a rehabilitation department in Marlborough, Massachusetts, said, "The director must have the personality to empower those who work for them, and to think out of the box and deliver."

Food and dietary services: *When a patient is admitted to a facility, assigned a room, and meets the staff and the doctor, the first questions usually are, "When is the next meal? Where is it served? What will it be? Can I change it?" You will know the cafeteria is good if the meals are varied, plentiful, and of good quality.*

During your walk through the facility, it is essential to either visit the kitchen or see a meal being sent to a resident. You can tell just by the look and smell that an investment has been made to serve each patient's dietary needs. It would be helpful to ask when the food services close for the night and whether the cafeteria provides snacks between meals.

You must follow the correct dietary orders. The department's food selection is based on the food orders provided at admitting and changed as a patient's condition changes and improves. Scrutiny of what is on the plate is yours and your advocate's responsibility. Many things can happen to food orders in cooking and delivering the proper meal; mistakes can be made. **In some cases, they are deadly mistakes.**

Stacy D., my mother's niece, tells us, "I went to visit my grandmother at a hospital in Syracuse, New York. She was cognizant of everything around her and still possessed her wits. I stayed so she had company during dinner. The tray was delivered while we were chatting, and I noticed the food on her fork. It was poultry — on the fork and the plate. Grandma was highly allergic to any poultry, which would cause respiratory failure. I demanded a correction to the diet and replacement of the meal. If I had not been there as a visitor and advocate, she could have died."

You should review the composition of the meals during your walk-through. You or your advocate may want to schedule the walk-through just before or after mealtime. During my walk-through at the South Shore acute facility, the kitchen plates were taken to the patients' rooms. Therefore, I could quickly assess the lunch quality: chicken, mashed potatoes, and asparagus, all freshly cooked and with a pleasant smell.

My first transitional rehabilitation facility duration was four and a half months. The breakfast was "one muffin, a cup of coffee, orange juice, a milk, and a bowl of Wheaties." Other plates consisted of "powered eggs, one/two strips of bacon, coffee, juice, coffee, and Wheaties."

Unfortunately, it was not until my eighth SNF/post-acute facility outside Worcester, Massachusetts, that I received nutritious and genuine food.

The benefits of overlapping staff roles: Whether the rehabilitation facility is an acute or post-acute facility, it should have a policy or rule that "all staff offer to help each other."

Overlapping staff roles among medical professionals should not be compromised by outside commercial and corporate recommendations of *no* over-lapping staff roles.

"Studies have shown that role conflict and role ambiguity are big factors in work stress among organizations' employees. Since work stress is negatively related to job satisfaction, it is important to understand and alleviate role conflict and role ambiguity in organizations." (Vertech Technical University)

Each organization has its way of educating new medical professionals about its mission statement, code of conduct, and residents' rights. First, you and your advocate should see such documents on the facility's walls, brochure, or website. Then, you should add that criterion to your checklist during the walk-through and interview.

Overlapping staff roles at a medical institution is a must for appropriate patient attention. This book has defined many staff roles you will find at a hospital or rehabilitation facility. The medical professionals generally on the floor with you are the nurse practitioners, RNs, CNAs, OT, PT, orderlies, and maintenance. **When interviewing, you should ask whether the medical professionals work overlapping and help each other work for the patient's benefit.**

An excellent example of a lack of teamwork is the call light outside your room. Should the staff refuse to work as a team, your call's response will be compromised.

During my first extended stay at a rehabilitation organization, it became apparent that no one would respond to the call light after I pressed the call button. The situation was so blatant that it became necessary to wheelchair myself into the hallway. There were two night nurses and two orderlies on the floor during the night shift, but no one responded to the call light. I had to go to the nurse's station in my wheelchair and ask for my pain meds and a drink. The orderlies were asleep in the common area.

It was not until I went to the facility outside Worcester, Massachusetts, that the staff overlapped. If the call light was on, the company's policy was "the first staff member to see the light must respond immediately. If the person nearest your room could not respond, that staffer was required to communicate the need to the next-closest staff member."

Staff working together can accommodate your needs, such as helping you get in and out of bed, the wheelchair, or calling the cafeteria. Whatever the requirement, the time to respond is cut to a minimum if staff overlap their roles. The policy at my facility was in writing: "NO employee should ever pass a room with a call light on!"

To assure yourself that overlapping does occur at the three facilities you select, ask for the actual mission statement and pages from the certified nursing assistants' training manual. Ensure overlap is a policy of the rehabilitation guidelines stated in a nurse's manual. This is an example: "It is the expectation that NO employee should ever pass a room with a call bell light on, without stopping in to ask the resident if they can be of assistance. The individual responding first 'owns' the request from the resident."

The orientation book requires anyone to respond to the call bell and communicate the resident's needs to the appropriate person. The conduct pertains to nurses, CNAs, doctors, and non-licensed professionals.

You may want to ask to see the "Dignity Code of Conduct." Dignity is essential for your respect. The code mentions privacy in the room, soiled clothes, food spillage, stained clothing, and grooming.

Having been a resident in both bad and good facilities, I understand that these codes are significant for you. When medical professionals overlap their roles and follow mission statements, your rehabilitation will have the best chance of restoring your health.

In earlier sections, I mentioned that a facility had a ratio of one CNA on a floor of 20 patients. **Here is when the question of ratios is essential.**

Safety of the facility and staff for the patient: *Each facility must be investigated by the state for your safety to limit the possibility you could hurt yourself.*

I was new to such places and did not have the opportunity for an onsite visit before being sent to my first rehab facility. The building had three floors. The first floor was for dementia care, the second floor for orthopedic care and other illnesses, and the third floor was assigned for long-term patients.

On the third floor resided a man with a long-term illness. He was an alcoholic named Jack. He would wait for the night shift to come on duty. Then he would dress in civilian clothes, take the elevator to the first floor, make sure the office person was gone or busy, walk out of the facility, buy a bottle at the liquor store, and then return.

There was no monitoring of patient rooms, the elevator codes were always the same, and the front door was always unlocked. Safety was not a priority for that organization, which was dangerous for the patients.

In two other physical rehabilitation facilities where I stayed, the facility clarified its patient safety responsibilities and rules. The rules are in place to not hurt yourself or others. An example is having a CNA or staff walk you to the bathroom if your condition requires, so you do not fall. Another safety rule is not to allow a patient to use a device, such as a walker if the patient is not authorized and trained to use it.

Safety goes both ways. The facility must comply with safety regulations from the state and the facility's management. When a nurse, CNA, or volunteer comes to the facility or hospital, they must have had appropriate training, including safety for you and themselves. Here is an excerpt from a safety regulation in the training manual on Caregiver Prevention Efforts:

- Check all residents at the beginning of all shifts.
- Check all seatbelts, alarms, and other safety devices at the start of your shift.
- Answer call lights and alarms quickly.
- Immediately clean up spills.
- Never leave a resident unattended in the bathroom if you assisted him/her into the bathroom.

There are authorities you can talk to if you feel continually unsafe. The head nurse, nursing director, and facility director are the first to contact for help. Then there are independent or state authorities where you can report your troubles. One such organization is the Joint Commission of Health and Safety. This is how you and other patients can report:

08/23/2018

"Beginning September 1, consumers reporting patient safety concerns will be directed to share the information exclusively online. It has always been our policy to receive reports about patient safety events in writing. Submitting these reports online is more direct and, importantly, helps our office act more quickly." (08/23/2018 jointcommission.org)

The Joint Commission; phone: 800-994-6610; fax: 630-792-5636; email: complaint@jointcommission.org: Office of Quality Monitoring, The Joint Commission, One Renaissance Boulevard, Oakbrook Terrace, IL 60181

Cautionary signs at an "onsite visit" of the rehabilitation facility

Cleanliness: You should be able to see if there is clutter in the hallways, a bathroom with stains or droppings, unkempt beds, dirty furniture, or common areas with trash or fluid stains.

Everyday essentials: Features that provide comfort and relaxation during your stay should be convenient: a TV that is easy to view and change channels; space that is large enough to use a wheelchair or crutches; bathroom doors that are wide enough for wheelchairs and space with accessible grab bars; and maneuverable meal trays.

Hallway and smells: One of the first genuine evaluations of a rehabilitation facility is the smell in the air and people sitting in the hallways. The smell of urine tells you a great deal about cleanliness. The staff must move patients out of their rooms, but urinating will occur when they sit and sleep for an extended period. You must consider such as environment as unacceptable and a sign of potential neglect.

Even in the current no-smoking era, smoking might be a necessary activity for the patient who is addicted to cigarettes. Investigate whether patients can smoke outside and when. If there are lines at the patio doors, you may want to rethink the stay. It is good to judge the patients who form lines at the door. Notice the clothes they are wearing.

I visited one of the post-acute care facilities I had stayed at in the past. After interviewing the new facility director, we walked through the hallway where patients had lined up to go out to the patio and smoke. The dirty language and dirty clothes raised a red flag for me, and the smell of smoke radiated through the hallway. I said, "Those people do not look sick or ill." The director's response was, "We have patients who are homeless and covered by government insurance. They need to be off the streets because of illnesses they might have or for safety reasons since they are homeless."

The physical and occupational therapy service area: A facility with only parallel bars, simulated bed, simulated stairs, agility balls, a small room, and a bike signals negative healthcare.

I was naive about the equipment and occupational tools necessary for good rehabilitation for five of my stays. Ask the tour guide and administrator whether physical and occupational therapists are employees or contractors. Cutting costs could account for lack of tools and a contractor's presence. On the other hand, hiring a contractor or outside service may mean the therapist requires billable hours. They may take you out of your room and wheel you to the PT area, even though you cannot perform therapy activity.

I have seen therapists take a patient off the bed and into a wheelchair while the man was crying and resisting because he had soiled his diaper with diarrhea.

The absence of recreation and hairdressing departments:

> **The recreation department:** A significant contributor to a healthy stay and taking your mind off medical procedures and pain is the recreation department. If the surgeon and the nurse practitioner feel your stay will be more than four days and there is no recreation department, you will have plenty of free time. Free time without activity leads to boredom, loneliness, and depression.

I met Steve and Paul during two of my stays at the facility outside Worcester, Massachusetts. Steve had a knee infection, and Paul a hip infection. Both men required skilled nursing for six weeks before their aspiration tests. It was their first stay at a skilled rehabilitation facility, and each of them was bored, complaining, and unhappy. I insisted they come with me to the recreation function. Both Steve and Paul became the most popular recreation patients in the facility. Before his discharge, **Steve commented to me that "the recreation kept me busy; I forgot the pain and it cheered me up for four weeks."**

Should your stay be longer than four days, recreation must be a vital consideration in your choice of a rehab facility.

Recreation for long-term residents is essential. Most of the rehabilitation brochures have the words "long-term residents." These are residents who will be there for the rest of their lives or until they no longer understand where they are. In some shape or form, recreation will provide a spark of love and humanity to their last days. You should not consider sharing recreation with long-term residents as unfavorable. Your short-term contribution to the experience of meeting them could fill your heart with joy forever.

During my last four stays in Millbury, I befriend three ladies playing bingo who were long-term residents: Cat, Jane, and Chris. We would laugh, talk, and compete against the other players. But, best of all, we appreciated each other's company and forgot about where we were and the pain we were in.

There are few things more rewarding, no matter what stage of illness, than hearing the resident yell "Bingo!!"

The need for hairdressing: Whether your man or a woman, feeling good about yourself and being refreshed is synonymous with getting your hair washed, cut, and styled. Hairdressers are built into our social culture. Even if the building has a contracted hairdresser, enjoyment is the same. You should add "access to a wash and cut" as a bonus on your checklist for choosing that SNF.

Recreation and access to a haircut are beneficial to you in acute and post-acute facilities. As a patient and then a volunteer at the Millbury facility, I witnessed women and men lined up for hair care an hour before the salon opened. The most rewarding outcome for the visitors, the staff, and other patients is the patients' glow when complimented on their hair. **Investing in a salon at a facility generates smiles all around.**

Conduct that interferes with your care:

Disagreement with insurance: I have spoken to several families and advocates, confident that a relative/friend was not ready to leave the rehabilitation facility. The RNs and physical therapists agreed that further rehabilitation was necessary, but the insurance company disagreed. If that happens, you or your advocate must speak up. You, your family or advocate, and your caregivers know your needs and limits; the insurance company does not.

John was informed that his insurance moved up his discharge with only a two-day notice. The insurance company explained that the daily rehabilitation reports received from the facility stated that he had walked farther than 100 feet. The fact that John walked 100 feet was the indicator that it was time for discharge in their policies for his illness. Thus, the responsibility fell upon John, his daughter, and his wife to prove the case for more rehabilitation. The hospital staff helped back up the family by submitting reports confirming that John needed more care.

It is a very emotional rollercoaster ride when the hospital or SNF has a conversation with you, your family, or your advocate relaying premature discharge. The following organizations may help.

> "Medicare beneficiaries and their advocates who question the appropriateness of a proposed discharge from a Medicare hospital, whether the discharge is too soon or whether necessary post-hospital services are needed, should contact the local Quality Improvement Organization (QIO) and file a complaint. The beneficiary's hospital discharge notice should provide the name, address, and phone number of the QIO serving the hospital in question, along with instructions on how to file a complaint."
>
> (42 C.F.R. §§412.42-412.48)

Losing insurance through a patient's mistake: Whether you must go to an acute or post-acute rehabilitation facility, most rehabs have rules forbidding you to wander out of the facility. This may be due to insurance. You must know if the insurance looks at a person leaving the grounds of the facility as if they are "healthy enough to walk and travel, [so] insurance is not needed."

If a patient leaves without the facility's consent, the organization's insurance payments will stop. One of the nursing staff's roles is to create a report on your activity or lack of activity. That report will go to the administration to request payment from the insurance company. If you are not using the facility's services or have left the building and its grounds, the insurance company will be aware of your actions. (We are not talking about patients with dementia.)

Warning signs of inadequate care

An article by Kurtis Hiatt in *U.S. News and World Report* provides additional information about inadequate care signals in rehabilitation and long-term care. (https://health.usnews.com/health-news/best-nursing-homes/articles/2013/02/26/9-warning-signs-of-bad-care)

- Patients marked emotional and physical changes
- Unanswered and deflected questions
- Frantic, discordant, or inadequate staff
- High staff turnover
- Patient saying they do not want a specific staff person to care for them
- Constant ringing phones and unanswered call lights
- Dehydration and malnourishment
- Status quo reigns
- A bad feeling

The decision to go home

Releasing the patient: At an acute and post-acute care facility, patients are admitted with rehabilitation instructions. Those instructions vary by illness and the medical procedures you undergo in the hospital. Rehabilitation work is accomplished when the appropriate doctors, physical therapists, nurses, and social services have decided that your goals have been met and when it is safe for you to go home.

For example, you will be tested by physical and occupational therapy staff against your admission goals if you are recovering from stoke or orthopedic surgery. Once the directors of physical and occupational therapy sign off on your discharge, your paperwork will be sent to nursing, the floor doctor, the surgeon, and the administration. You will be informed about the next steps and your discharge planning.

You and the discharge team must mutually agree that all goals were met, and you can be discharged. Your surgery or illness is only one of many variables of recovery. Just because you have completed all the objectives does not mean changes will not be required at your home. Cooperation and being open to suggestions and new mobility practices are a must. I have seen patients and previous facility roommates dismiss follow-up care or home safety methods. A few had to go back to the hospital, and others had deadly falls. The bottom line is that you have new medical needs and must accept help and support.

When Dick had his quadruple bypass, discharge required input from the original surgeons, hospital departments, and rehabilitation staff. During the round-table consultations, home safety was at the top of the checklist. The topic of a home inspection surfaced. A home visit was required for his discharge. The facility staff went to Dick's house, checked for safety (clutter, no grab bars), made recommendations, and fulfilled the safety requirements before he could go home.

Allow social services and nursing to perform a walk-through of your residence. They will review safety, appropriate equipment, and follow-up home care for personal care concerns during the visit.

The National Institutes of Health (NIH) definition of discharge planning from a hospital in rehabilitation facility, and skilled nursing facilities is "the development of a discharge plan for follow-up services for a patient before leaving the hospital [to contain] costs, and improv[e] patient outcomes. Discharge planning is a complex process, and many healthcare disciplines may contribute to the plan, including formal discharge planning coordinators, nurses, social workers, physical therapists, occupational therapists, and physicians.

"Reviews of discharge planning processes showed that they consistently involve the assessment of many factors, including cognitive, physical, social/financial status, environmental concerns, and access to formal and informal care."

Usually, a final consultation and signature are required for release to the family and/or advocate. Then, you will be taken home by the family, or the facility logistics manager will arrange transportation. The logistics manager will call for transport by ambulance with the appropriate accommodations for a safe ride home.

Acquiring therapy tools for home use: At the time of discharge, you must have the appropriate tools to use at home for your therapy and safety. The hospital or rehabilitation facility's physical therapy specialist will discuss the necessary items. Due to your therapy at the facility, you should be proficient in using these tools before leaving. They can be wheelchairs, canes, walkers, grabbers, sock helpers, lifts, shower chairs, hand or grab bars (used to help get off the toilet, chair, or bed), shoe assistants, etc.

Some helpful suggestions include:

- Insurance should pay for some tools that can be taken home from the hospital or rehabilitation facility. Ask the administrator.
- Senior centers in your city or town will have items that have been donated by others who no longer require their use.
- Medical supply stores often honor your insurance.
- Websites like Craigslist.com, Nextdoor.com, Amazon, or Facebook Marketplace may have listings about tools available at a small cost, but it is critical to sterilize these before using them.
- Let It Go offers used items from providers close to your home.

When I required crutches to move around, I found it impossible to use my hands to carry anything. For example, I went to my local drugstore to get medicine and other products, but I could not carry them without a backpack. I had the same problem with a bottle of soda/water. So, I searched Amazon for crutch helpers and found side pockets attached to the crutch frame using Velcro straps. They hold bottles, cellphones, newspapers, and other daily living products. The crutch holders made home recovery far more manageable.

Using tools after coming home can be difficult and embarrassing for a time. The fact is that you are your advocate. Do what you must do to heal.

Home Care

The web defines home health nursing as a "nursing specialty in which nurses provide multidimensional home care to patients of all ages. Home health care is a cost-efficient way to deliver quality at the client's home's convenience. Home health nurses create care plans to achieve goals based on the client's diagnosis."

The people committed to home care have a unique skill set, including knowing and understanding care management needs for acute and chronic illnesses and disabilities. They are experts at leading teams to help you be as functional as possible or manage new disabilities. They will monitor, review, and evaluate outcomes while focusing on quality care and achieving milestones. In addition, home care nurses fully understand the resources available at each level of Post-Acute Care (PAC).

I contacted three home rehabilitation companies for four separate operations. However, it is one thing to have acute, post-acute, and hospital care, where there are other patients and dozens of medical professionals nearby. It is an entirely different matter when you are home and alone. You are assigned a caregiver who will need to make it through every day; do not be humiliated. They have your best interest in mind and will do the required job. They also will be proficient with your medical devices and medicine.

When questioning whether to go home, the surgeon and nurse practitioner are the best people to answer these questions: "Do I need rehab? How can the caregiver help me? How long should I expect them to stay?"

Be aware: The hospital medical professionals will avoid answering the question, "Which home care company should I chose?"

Should you insist on home care when that choice differs from the surgeon's suggestion, you must determine whether the insurance company will cover home care of any kind. For example, the insurance company may insist on the surgeon's recommendation for release to home care. Once confirmed, the medical professionals will verify that the home has been equipped with therapy tools to prevent a fall and has appropriate safety measures (level floor, no stairs, and sufficient space to move around).

(https://www.medicare.gov/homehealthcompare/compare.html#cmprTab=1&cmprID=227596%2C227479&stsltd=MA&loc=01581&lat=42.2638905&lng=-71.6080009)

It is crucial to have medical professionals working with you to offer multiple recovery activities. Be patient and cooperative. Being disruptive with the therapy could invalidate your insurance.

Short-Term Home Care and Preparation: Medline Plus.gov defines short-term care as care that is "required for a couple of days to a few months. Like long-term care, short-term care can be provided in a variety of settings. This includes a hospital, an assisted living facility, a nursing home residence, and one's home."

Home care companies offer varied short-term services to smooth the transition from the hospital to your home. However, should you be released directly from the hospital to home care or spend weeks in a physical rehabilitation care facility, you might still experience pain and mental trauma. The nurses dispatched by the home care providers must know the extent of your medical procedures to address this. Once armed with that information, a nurse will have the qualifications to evaluate and arrange the home care service personnel to work best with you.

Preparing for short-term home care: If you have had an extensive and intrusive operation, home care is likely to be necessary. If you are sent to an acute care facility and without time to formulate a plan, you and your advocate should be able to investigate options while you are in acute care. Otherwise, the hospital social worker and facility social worker can help you.

Home care covered all eleven of my recovery needs. The companies worked similarly, whether it pertained to the spine, knee, hips, heart, or renal system.

- The patient, hospital, or advocate must select one home care company even if it sends nurses to the home for a short time. Usually, there is no onsite meeting; the discussions will be over the phone or face-to-face at home using computer vision software.
- An agenda must include insurance coverage through primary and secondary policies. Geographic coverage is essential. Check that your insurance covers them and you are within their home care covered area.
- The nurse in charge will visit the home, check vital signs such as blood pressure, take a close look at the wound or acute status and discuss everything relevant to your care. Examples would be attitude, pain level, mobility, equipment, and mental outlook. A schedule for ongoing visits will be set up.

  I was alone for all my operations and interviewed the nurses and home care providers myself. A family member or advocate is essential in these critical times if you can arrange for them to be present or on the phone.

- The nurse reports back to the organization, and a home health caregiver is assigned. The process begins.

I suggest requesting a hospital representative and HMO person be assigned to your home recovery. They will provide a direct link to the doctors, at least by phone.

After my knee operation, the home care nurse, while checking the wound with her hand, found two stitches not removed by the rehabilitation facility. I had to go back to the surgeon for their removal. The surgeon told me that if the home care nurse had not been there to investigate the wound, "Infection might have set in." It would be best to welcome nurse orientation visits and home health caregivers. Work with them. They often notice things that no one else has.

Long-Term Home Care: The National Institute of Aging says that "home-based long-term care includes health, personal, and support services to help people stay at home and live as independently as possible. Most long-term care is provided either in the home of the person receiving services or at a family member's home."

Long-term services are generally for people with chronic and progressive conditions, such as Parkinson's disease, a debilitating stroke, renal failure, Alzheimer's disease, dementia, or kidney failure requiring dialysis. In these instances, consistent assistance and care are a must. "If somebody needs help over the long term, the question is, 'Are those needs going to remain relatively consistent or will they increase?'" says Val Halamandaris, president of the National Association for Home

Care & Hospice. "If the situation is becoming more complex, you will need to add more services gradually."

"Most family members have no experience or training in caring for a chronically ill person at home. Bathing mom or dad is one thing, but changing a colostomy bag, suctioning secretions from a tracheotomy tube, or monitoring a ventilator is more than most family caregivers can safely take on. [For] in-home dialysis, a preplanned process is required for the home caregiver; they may be overwhelmed. In these cases, you should hire skilled home care on a long-term basis until the [patient]'s needs exceed what can be provided in the home. Around-the-clock supervision and higher levels of care and training may become necessary. Services usually conclude when the elder moves to an assisted living facility or nursing home." (National Association of Home Care and Hospice)

This is a story from Carmen S. of Westborough, Massachusetts. Carmen details what transpired with her husband, Mark. The story is important because you will learn about the system of critical home care, training for around-the-clock home care, and when the responsibility is too much to handle. Although the healthcare system attempts to provide solutions to managing care at home, it can fail due to the human factor. **The medical system, the family, and the advocate need to know when to say "no."**

"My husband had multiple diagnoses. He battled Stage 4 kidney disease and neuropathy. His kidney doctor insisted that we were 'good candidates' for home dialysis treatment on a bedside dialysis machine.

"What made us viable in the doctor's view? We both were retired from high-tech sales careers and trained to introduce new business processes and solutions — but we never imagined that taking on the required levels of human, environmental, and medical care would debilitate us with mental fatigue and physical burnout in a matter of weeks! Yet, even with the help of nurses who visited our home weekly or needed, it happened.

"When my husband's kidneys failed in mid-August 2019, his prescribed home dialysis was accelerated with little time to learn new required processes or become familiar with daily medical routines. As a result, we had to prepare a complicated schedule to implement:

"Home storage of 60 cases: dialysis solution and medical supplies (gloves, masks, sterile bandages) and set up a monthly schedule for replenishment.

"Rearrange/move treatment room (master bedroom) furniture to accommodate dialysis machine, solution set-up table, supplies table; create space for wheelchair weighing machine and hanging solution stand (required in the event of a power outage for manual dialysis). Create a sterile clean treatment room/bathroom environment — daily wipe-downs for the machine, washing bedding/clothes, dusting/vacuuming, preparing hand-washing station (cleaners, paper towels, gloves, masks).

"Arrange a schedule for a two-member nursing team to arrive at home for two weeks at 7 a.m. to initiate home dialysis class with flip charts, manuals, regular quizzes, and a final exam to take responsibility as a primary caregiver.

"Learn daily, sterile stomach catheter exit-wound care: sterilize site, apply antibiotic cream, apply new dressings.

"Perform and record daily monitoring of Mark's weight, blood pressure, temperature, and dialysis solution amounts. Schedule solution exchange samples every three weeks for dialysis clinic checkups.

"As the primary caregiver, I arranged training (supervised by the nursing team member) for a back-up caregiver in the event of illness or burnout.

"Monthly clinic meeting for doctor consult, bloodwork testing, vaccine shots, hemoglobin infusions (if needed), and prescription/menu reviews.

"Make frequent (weekly) dietary adjustments to keep chemical body elements (electrolytes) in proper balance, requiring new supplements, food items, or medicines.

"Within three weeks of nurses coming and going, treatment area cleaning, food/supplement shopping, laundry, phone calls, plus dialysis machine alarms on average of two hours every night because 'the solution line was blocked,' I became emotionally overwhelmed! Four weeks from the start of home dialysis, Mark's heart failed.

"What could have been done to scope out and implement these complicated duties better? What questions were not asked? What processes were not detailed? What caregiver side-effects were not addressed? Never in my life had I felt more inadequate to help the one I so wanted to help – my husband of 31 years!

"It is my opinion, in-depth discussions in advance on the following topics would have helped me prepare for the realities of this life-saving treatment:

"1. Importance of sterile/clean treatment environments and maintaining them.

"2. Nuances of maintaining/operating dialysis machine/ clearing frequent alarms.

"3. Ways to prevent/reduce the chance of burnout, warning signs.

"4. Identify/confirm back-up caregiver well in advance of the start date.

"5. Deeper knowledge of chemical body elements and a list of foods to balance body requirements.

"6. Understanding that home dialysis becomes the #1 priority in your life – all other activity is re-prioritized around this daily treatment discipline.

"7. The effects of dialysis on the body and how to mitigate them.

"8. At what point should I have asked for another level of care?

"I provided 'institutionalized' medical care in our master bedroom, which was transformed into a quasi-medical clinic. The decision to proceed is life-altering and must be done with 'eyes wide open.'

"If my experiences can help another considering this type of care, then all is not lost. I send you my support and understanding."

Whether it is short-term or long-term home care, every element of the process must be understood, so you are assured that you follow what was prescribed and can safely handle the circumstances.

To recap, if the surgeons and your primary doctor feel home recovery, home nursing, and outpatient physical therapy are best for your condition, there must be due diligence before the home care experience. **Questions need to be asked and answered.**

COVID-19: Hospital and rehabilitation decisions: The COVID-19 pandemic means that you and your family may need to be prepared if you have to send or deliver a loved one to a hospital. Use the decision-making techniques described above for hospitals and rehabilitation facilities. Use the websites in each section to choose a facility for battling COVID-19. Deciding on a surgeon will not be relevant in COVID-19 cases other than being referred to a hospital.

Note: Before going to a hospital, secure your preferred hospital using Carmen S.'s technique. You can also join the CDC through their website.

Carmen S. had stayed several times at Union Hospital in Framingham, Massachusetts. Still, if she had shown acute symptoms of COVID-19 quickly and called an ambulance, the Westborough ambulance service would have been required to go to the nearest hospital that could treat the illness. That would be UMass Worcester, where she did not want to go. Knowing that preference in advance, Carmen performed due diligence on UMass and Union Hospital before the virus revealed its symptoms.

The only way Carmen could be admitted to Union Hospital's emergency room of her choice was to get her transportation and not call 911 for an ambulance. Armed with that information, Carmen recruited two advocates who would take her to Framingham. The advocates she spoke with, having learned about the issue of choice, recruited their advocates to implement Carmen's technique for a hospital of choice.

<u>If your symptoms are severe, do what is good for your health and safety: Call 911.</u>

Preparation for your care: Combating COVID-19 is a living process we all need to battle. Although vaccines are available, mutations of COVID-19 will develop over time. Therefore, procedures will change continuously, but much of what you read now can still be applied as virus prevention, care, and cures moving forward.

Symptom categories and statistics: Once you start to develop any of the following symptoms, get tested. Let your medical professional at a hospital or your primary doctor suggest whether you can safely stay at home. Hartford Healthcare grouped symptoms by percentages for easier self-diagnosis (May 5, 2020).

"Initial COVID-19 symptoms vary, but the Centers for Disease Control and Prevention says most people with a coronavirus infection will experience:

- Fever (83–99 percent)
- Cough (59–82 percent)
- Fatigue (44–70 percent)
- Anorexia/loss of appetite (40–84 percent)
- Shortness of breath (31–40)
- Sputum production (28–33 percent)
- Muscle aches (11–35 percent)"

As of July 2020, stated that www.CDC.gov had added:

- Runny nose
- Sore throat
- Congestion
- Nausea
- Diarrhea
- Abnormal behavior

Critical symptoms — hospital decision time: The CDC suggests emergency attention when the following signs become consistent or acute.

"Look for emergency warning signs (of COVID-19). If someone is showing any of these signs, seek emergency medical care immediately:

- Trouble breathing
- Persistent pain or pressure in the chest
- New confusion
- Inability to wake or stay awake
- Bluish lips or face

This symptom list is not complete. Call your medical provider if any other symptoms that are severe or concerning to you."

Responsibility of the COVID-19 homecare giver: As of now, home caregivers have not become responsible for providing more advanced medical devices, such as respirators, at home. The training, devices, and amount of work that Carmen S. experienced are not authorized or recommended by medical professionals.

The CDC recommends actions for a home care individual who has COVID-19 and the caregiver:

"If you are caring for someone with COVID-19 at home or in a non-healthcare setting, follow this advice to protect yourself and others. Learn what to do when someone has symptoms of COVID-19 or when someone has been diagnosed with the virus. This information also should be followed when caring for people who have tested positive but are not showing symptoms. (https://www.cdc.gov/coronavirus/2019-ncov/if-you-are-sick/care-for-someone.html)

Note: Older adults and people of any age with underlying severe medical conditions are at higher risk of developing more severe illness from COVID-19 or mutant viruses. Anyone at higher risk of severe disease should call their doctor as soon as symptoms are identified.

The caregiver will support and help to cover basic needs:

- See whether over-the-counter medicines for fever reduce the temperature.
- Help the sick person follow their doctor's instructions for care and meds. For most people, symptoms last a few days, and people usually feel better after a week.
- Remind the person who is sick to drink fluids and rest.
- Help with grocery shopping and filling prescriptions. Consider having items delivered.
- Help with pet care and limit the time between the sick person and their pet(s).
- Get their doctor's phone number.
- Use CDC's self-checker tool to help make decisions in seeking appropriate medical care.
- Call their doctor if the person keeps getting sicker. For medical emergencies, call 911 and tell the dispatcher that the person has or might have COVID-19."

Protecting yourself when caring for a COVID-19 patient:
https://www.cdc.gov/coronavirus/2019-ncov/prevent-getting-sick/prevention.html

- Limit contact.
- Eat in another room.

- Avoid sharing items.
- Wear a face cover and gloves.
- Wash your hands often.
- Clean and disinfect the house, bathroom, and bedroom.
- Wash and dry laundry after every use.
- Use lined trash bags.
- Check your health.

Hope — Fight — Live: No matter how minor or complicated a process and surgery might be, any procedure can be problematic. Your role is to Hope — Fight — Live.

All diagnoses must be taken seriously for the illness to be eliminated. Hope allows you to hold on. The fight is working your courage and commitment. Work the process as a team member, convinced that your strength would make a good quality of life happen. Live against all odds. **Should a simple procedure cause an infection, organs become weaker, or cancer comes back, you should strive to overcome it all and live so some essence of quality of life is achieved.**

By being proactive, you can change your lifestyle to prevent the severe illnesses mentioned above that put you in the high-risk category and feeding COVID-19.

As Doctor Edward Hoffer wrote on page 95 of *Prescription for Bankruptcy*, "differences in lifestyle, eating habits, exercise, and culture all play a role. The *Journal of Circulation* in April 2018 found that five healthy behaviors could add twelve to fourteen years to the life span of middle-aged adults: a healthy diet, regular exercise, not smoking, maintaining a healthy weight, and moderate intake of alcohol. These factors were associated with a reduced rate of cancer, cardiovascular disease, and overall mortality."

CHAPTER THREE

PAIN AND COMMUNICATION

The Oxford Dictionary definition of pain is:
"*Noun* – physical suffering or discomfort caused by illness or injury."

The definition of pain used by *Medicinenet* is:
"An unpleasant sensation that can range from mild, localized discomfort to agony ... The physical part of pain results from nerve stimulation. Your pain may be contained in a discrete area. Similar/synonyms – agony; affliction; torture; torment; discomfort."

Pain! Pain has reached out and touched me due to spine infections, hip infections, and neuropathy. During a good part of these experiences, I had no pain medicine, and unfortunately, friends and doctors did not believe me about the extent of the pain.

Since I had been healthy most of my life, they assumed, "He has something that will pass, or it could be in his head." It was not until I called Don Hanssen and begged for help that my friends started to take me seriously. Don and Mike Garrison took me to Mike's house in Canton, Massachusetts. The reality of the agony became apparent when Mike found me on the floor in a fetal position, trying to adjust my body to take the pressure off the sciatic nerve.

What I experienced was a social problem called "pain stigma." It pertains to circumstances when a person or patient's affliction, matching the definition above, is not taken seriously. You may experience pain stigma at some time in your life. Therefore, you must understand how to communicate your pain to medical professionals effectively.

Pain is relative to those who experience it. Pain can have a short duration and can be intermittent, acute, or chronic. Chronic pain extends over a long time. An example of a short course of pain is a woman delivering a baby without medication. Patients with cancer or burn victims endure chronic pain for an extended period.

Many of the individuals who provided testimonials for this book suffered long-lasting pain from war wounds, non-correctable orthopedic deformities, cancer, infections, and nerve damage.

Pain is relative to the patient: As Ivan R. Molton, Ph.D., states in "Assessing Pain," "Feelings of pain and pain-related suffering are personal and internal events. Although certain body systems may change in response to pain, there is no biological marker for pain, and there is no blood test or other objective measurement to determine how much pain a person is in, or how much that pain is affecting her or him. For that reason, virtually all pain assessment is based on subjective self-reporting."

If pain should be self-reporting, the patient must assess and communicate pain through approved multiple measurement tools. For instance, Kim O'Brien stated, "The 0 to 10 pain scale was useless." She told surgeons that her pain was Level 2 and mild, so they dismissed her situation as minimal and did nothing. The result of this miscommunication led to wrong decisions by doctors.

I am supportive of pain scales. Learning the pain intensity during each infection helped me set a baseline for pain and determine my intense pain level. However, Kim O'Brien should have been asked more questions to make the doctor uncover why she experienced dizziness, her legs were numb, and she was falling. Those questions might have led to further tests and scans.

Communication with doctors may require multiple-dimensional tools. There are three proven techniques to bring to doctors at the first or second consultation. Understand that these suggestions are for both the physician and the patient. Be prepared to be your self-advocate.

Clinical interviewing of symptoms and mild pain: The doctor can ask open-ended questions about your ability and behavior. Kim could not express pain through the pain level scale. Her skills and actions were the keys that the surgeon needed to focus on. "Open questions" could have been asked of her. Be prepared to answer or ask questions at every surgeon consultation; be your advocate. Ivan Molton, a researcher of pain, uses the following questions to determine pain level.

- How do the numbness and dizziness affect your normal daily activities?
- Is there pain when these symptoms occur?
- How does the problem affect your emotions and state of mind?
- Do you sleep well?
- Can other people see your symptoms as they occur?

In 2010, Doctor Molton adapted six topics from renowned scientists and researchers of pain (Dennis C. Turk, James P. Robinson, and Tasha Burwinkle, Department of Anesthesiology, University of Washington, Seattle, Washington). Their studies showed that you should answer these topics and communicate the medical professional's answers during the consultation: How dizziness, pain in the stomach, fainting, or pain in the hips and knees work with your intensity, activities, coping, thoughts, upset, and how other people see you during the discomfort.

1. **Intensity:** Is this a change from your usual level of pain? Rate the severity of your pain now.
2. **Activities:** How does the pain affect your ability to sleep, eat, and be active?
3. **Coping:** What relievers lessen your pain?
4. **Thoughts:** What are your thoughts about pain? Do you think you will always have pain?
5. **Upset:** Does your pain cause feelings of fear, worry, anxiety, or depression?

6. **People:** How do others react when you are in pain, and how do their reactions affect you?

In Kim O'Brien's case, her pain was irrelevant. Instead, her symptoms should have led to multiple testing. Her "incapability" should have been recognized and diagnosed by the first two specialty surgeons she saw.

Use of multiple pain level scales: Don Hanssen and Mike Garrison took me to see an orthopedic surgeon at their local hospital. After ordering an X-ray, MRI, and CT scan, the surgeon's comment was, "Mr. Butler, your left hip has disintegrated." He asked what activities I could do and whether I was emotional or depressed. I replied that I was incapable of climbing stairs, sleeping, and killing the pain with alcohol. Alcohol made me depressed and was habit-forming. My answers indicated that pain was the primary symptom and that chemicals or painkillers were ineffective. My former lifestyle was gone, and I was incapable of withstanding any more pain.

A more detailed description of measuring pain came from www.prohealth.com and is included below. Refer to the descriptions of your symptoms and match them to your pain level when communicating with your primary doctor, specialists, post-operative staff, and rehabilitation facility staff and during recovery appointments.

The objective is for you and the medical professional to speak the same language.

"It is crucial that you take the pain scale seriously.

Because pain is subjective, it is difficult to explain what you feel to another person — even your doctor. To effectively use the pain scale, familiarize yourself with the levels before your procedure, identifying what key levels indicate your pain level. Following surgery or procedure, typically, we tell patients to continue to take medications that allow them to maintain a level of '5 or below.'

0 — Pain-Free

Mild Pain — *Nagging, annoying, but does not interfere with daily living activities.*
1 — Pain is very mild, barely noticeable. Most of the time, you do not think about it.
2 — Minor pain. It annoying and may have occasional stronger twinges.
3 — Pain is noticeable and distracting; however, you can get used to it and adapt.

Moderate Pain — *Interferes significantly with daily living activities.*
4 — Moderate pain. If you are deeply involved in an activity, it can be ignored for a period; but still distracting.
5 — Moderately severe pain. You cannot ignore it for more than a few minutes, but you can still manage to work or participate in some social activities with effort.
6 — Moderately severe pain that interferes with regular daily activities. I cannot concentrate.

Severe Pain — *Disabling; unable to perform daily living activities.*
7 — Severe pain that dominates your senses and significantly limits your ability to perform routine daily activities or maintain social relationships. Interferes with sleep.
8 — Intense pain. Physical activity is severely limited. Conversing requires great effort.
9 — Excruciating pain. Unable to converse. Crying out and moaning uncontrollably.
10 — Unspeakable pain. Bedridden and possibly delirious. Significantly few people will ever experience this level of pain."

In her book *A Patient's Perspective*, Patricia Cyr says, "I think a scale of 1 to 10 is a poor tool for assessing chronic conditions whose symptoms are variable. Sometimes I might write, for example, that my pain varies from a 2 to 8. Practitioners may not be happy about that, but it's the best I can offer."

Yes, all pain assessment is based on subjective self-reporting, but one must determine a pain level for chronic pain even if it is variable. In my case, the pain levels for the spine infections and hip infections started low — Level 2 — but gradually increased to between 7 and 9. Although it rose as time went on, the pain was always variable. Activities, body positions, standing, sitting, sleeping, and tools such as crutches varied the levels. There was chronic pain when the infections filled the tissue, and my bones and the broken stem of the prosthesis moved. The pain was variable but measurable when considered separately. I would set my pain levels at a base level relative to activities. As the pain became more intense, I would rate the pain higher relative to activity.

It would be best if you attempted to create a base and a high level of pain. The base-level can be established when pain is at its lowest and corresponds to the levels shown above. The higher level of pain you are experiencing matches the higher number above. There is a joke that goes, "The patient says, 'Doctor, it hurts when I do that.' The doctor says, 'Well, don't do that.'" Until the appropriate diagnosis has been verified by multiple specialists, "Don't do that." If the pain is chronic, you will know it, and then you must communicate to the medical professionals using the scale.

The pain scales shown have become an accepted way for people to rate their pain intensity. Using these descriptions, you can match the number on the scale to understand your illness.

The scales use words, images, or descriptors to communicate a measurement of pain to medical professionals. www.verywellhealth.com lists the standard unit-dimensional pain scales:

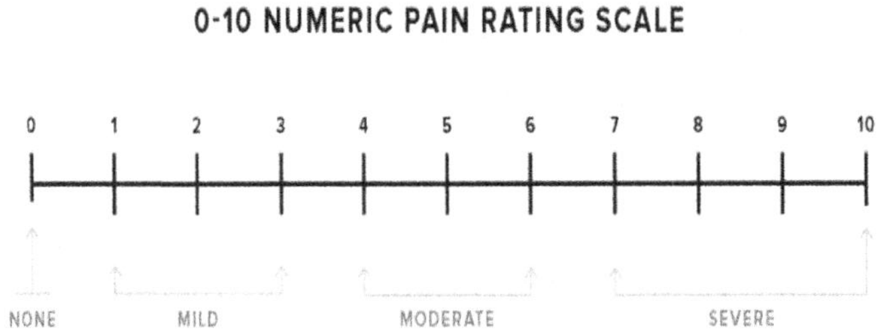

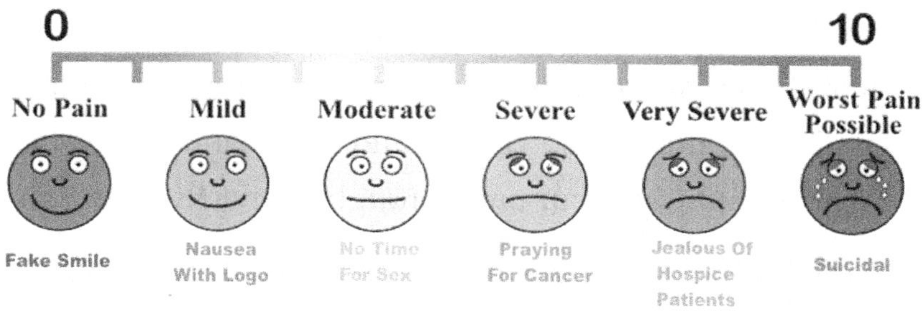

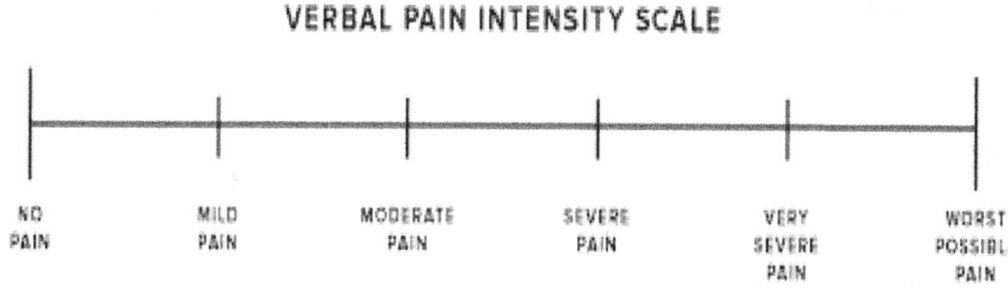

Other methods doctors and patients can use are:

1. Comfort Scale
2. Migill Scale
3. Color Analog Scale
4. Makoski Pain Scale
5. Brief Pain Inventory
6. Descriptor Differential Scale of Pain Intensity
7. FLACC Scale
8. Cries Scale

As I experienced variable pain levels in my hips over four years, I became incredibly good at communicating my baseline pain level and the chronic pain level when it varied. In every department or institution where I stayed, I was asked my pain level based on these scales.

The scales are an internationally used language you need to learn from the baseline (lowest number on the scale) to intense levels (higher numbers). You should learn and understand how to communicate your pain through your activities.

The astounding fact about human anatomy and recovery is how the body adapts during and after recovery. When I finally finished my last implant operation, the pain in my hips slowly diminished; even my spinal pain dropped.

While driving with Don Hanssen and his wife Ann, I commented that I could not remember or feel how bad the pain had been. Although the pain incapacitated my body, and I either yelled or cried at its peak, I could not remember the pain. Ann responded, "Bill, that is why women have more than one baby!" Her response was precious and authentic. The brain works to protect us from remembering pain and suffering.

Pain can be addressed by nature, drugs, activities, meditation, acupuncture, and lifestyle. Still, the fact is that you must be able to measure pain, identify your level, and know how to communicate that information to medical professionals.

> **Use of the word "Incapability" scale for symptoms:** She experienced the first major medical challenge in her life. She had not been educated, like most patients, about how to use the scale. She learned that symptoms and pain could be separate signals to the patient and the medical professional.

By replacing the word "pain" with the word "incapability" in the pain scale descriptions on www.prohealth.com, you may now be able to rate your level of capability and symptoms to your surgeon. The intent is to allow you to rate the symptoms' levels from your perspective. When I asked Kim to reevaluate herself using the Incapability Scale, she rated her illness severity from Level two to Levels 6 and 7. The descriptive levels of pain had not changed, and the internationally proven ratings had not changed. The only change was the word "incapability," relating to the severe symptoms with an apparent illness. **I created the "incapability" scale from Kim's experience and reworded it, so the scale is relative to "incapability."**

Let us see the difference it makes in communicating with medical professionals.

"It is important that you use the incapability scale for the symptoms you are experiencing."

Because incapability is subjective or may not exist in your case, it is difficult to explain what you feel to another person—even your doctor. Using the word "incapability," you can match the level of severity of your ability to function. Familiarize yourself with your level of incapability. Following surgery or procedure, typically, patients continue to be asked by medical professionals as they monitor their recovery.

0 – Incapability free

Mild incapability – Nagging, annoying, but does not interfere with daily living activities.

1 – Incapability's is mild, barely noticeable. Most of the time, you do not think about it.

2 — Minor incapability. Annoying and may have occasional stronger twinges.
3 — Incapability is noticeable and distracting; however, you can get used to it and adapt.

Moderate incapability — Interferes significantly with daily living activities.
4 — Moderate incapability. If you are deeply involved in an activity, it can be ignored for a period; but still distracting.
5 — Moderately strong incapability. You cannot ignore it for more than a few minutes, but you can still manage to work or participate in some social activities with the effort.
6 — Moderately strong incapability that interferes with regular daily activities. I cannot concentrate.

Severe incapability — Disabling; unable to perform daily living activities.
7 — Severe incapability that dominates your senses and significantly limits your ability to perform routine daily activities or maintain social relationships. Interferes with sleep.
8 — Intense incapability. Physical activity is severely limited. Conversing requires great effort.
9 — Excruciating incapability. Unable to converse. Crying out and moaning uncontrollably.
10 — Unbearable incapability. Bedridden and possibly delirious. Significantly few people will ever experience this level of incapability."

The descriptions above are just part of the overall consultation. Using more than one measurement scale should help identify your illness and allow the medical professional to make a more accurate diagnosis and testing.

Kim O'Brien was amazed to find that the descriptions matched the severity of her illness. "Replacing the word pain with the word 'incapability,' my levels would have been 6 and 7," she said. When I introduced this to her, she could clearly understand what she should have told the medical professionals. Medical professionals should have been more proactive and asked more detailed questions about her symptoms to assess her status.

Note: "The intangible "Incapacity Scale" described in this book is attributed to William Reiley Butler. This potential standard of measurement may assist in technological diagnoses. The concept, if future royalties should be applied, is protected by the Life's Realities, LLC and its author."

The stigma of pain: People often are, or feel they have been, the object of stigma because of debilitating pain. The *Oxford Dictionary* defines *stigma* as, "A mark branded on a criminal; or an imputation attaching to a person's reputation; a stain on one's good name." In "The relationship between mental disorder stigma interventions and individual differences," an unpublished master's thesis for the University of Calgary (2018), T. Neilson describes stigma as "a socially discredited attribute that causes rejection or discrimination, and outlines stigma's elements as labeling, stereotyping, separating, status loss, and discrimination."

The Institute for Chronic Pain defines stigma as "a significant and persistent problem for those with chronic pain. Stigma occurs when someone is judged for having a condition that they did not choose to have, like chronic pain. In other words, stigma is the criticism of being bad in some way for simply having a condition that you did not choose to have." (www.medicinenet.com).

The emotional effect of experiencing the stigma of pain is relative to the person receiving it. Unlike the pain scales, you cannot measure your impact, but it does exist. I have added this section in case you contract a disabling illness. **If you acknowledge stigma, friends, partners, business acquaintances, and loved ones may understand what harm they can do while admitting that you could be harming yourself.**

This section refers to those who have chronic pain, not those suffering from being a hypochondriac or having another mental illness. I break the stigma of pain into "self-stigma" and "social stigma." The intent is to help you understand this unfortunate problem because the impact of stigma can go both ways.

Daniel S. Goldberg, in an article about "Pain, objectivity, and history: understanding pain stigma" for BMJ talk medicine's "Health Justice with Dr. Oni Blackstock (January 23, 2020), says that "Pain does not stigmatize people. Instead, we do that to each other."

"Pain-related stigma can come from anyone," he wrote. "Health care providers are a major source of it, but so are intimate partners, family caregivers, insurers, and policymakers.

Chronic pain sufferers sometimes stigmatize other people with chronic pain, perhaps because of the difficulty of living with such a condition makes it harder to countenance in others, and people in pain sometimes stigmatize themselves. When you are told repeatedly that your pain is invalid or illegitimate, after a while, it becomes easy to believe that. People in pain do not have the luxury of denying the existence of their pain, but they can and do judge it."

Self-Stigma: P.W. Corrigan, J.E. Larson, and S.A. Kuwabara provide a helpful definition of self-stigma (2010) in J.E. Maddux and J.P. *Social psychology of the stigma of mental illness: Public and self-stigma models*. They said, "Self-stigmatization has been defined as the process in which a person with a mental health diagnosis becomes aware of public stigma, agrees with those stereotypes, and internalizes them by applying them to the self."

I use chronic pain and being disabled as the diagnosis, not a reference to mental health.

After my botched spine operation in 2011, I was incapacitated by a frail body and constant spinal pain. Even worse was the neuropathy in my right leg due to scar tissue from the additional three operations touching the nerves. After being active in numerous sports, such as tennis, martial arts, snow skiing, water skiing, hiking, and bowling, I now could not do any of them.

As time went on, my business partners, friends, and family recognized the difference in me. They slowly distanced themselves. The same thing happened five years later when both my hips became infected, and the pain was at its height. People will start to see you differently, which leads to social distancing, thus social stigma.

Remember Mark S., whose kidneys were failing? He was forced to engage others in his family only in the evenings because of medication and its effect on his morning and afternoon bodily functions. Others did not understand and backed away, stigmatizing him to stay home and venture out only occasionally. Thanks to his wife, Carmen, he maintained a positive attitude and believed that he was not alone due to a higher power. He controlled his pain and kept his self-worth. Mark won over self-stigma, right up to when he died.

When you cannot function as before and people's attitude toward you changes, you begin to internalize stigma. You start to lose hope and the ability to fight by thinking, "Am I overdramatizing? They are right. I do not need this medication. I do not try hard enough. I should just stay away from everyone and be by myself. I am crippled for the rest of my life. I cannot interview for a job anymore. I am a burden on everyone. It is all in my imagination." These negative thoughts ruin your motivation to move forward. You may lose hope.

An example of your friends and family's attitude changes can be as simple as excluding you from events because you show pain. People fear that your condition could happen to them; even worse, you may fall or have an episode and they are helpless of what to do or could be held liable.

For example, during my hip infections and double revision operations, I needed to use oxycodone to reduce pain so I could walk every morning. However, friends would lecture me about the negative aspects of the drug and tell me to use other pain reduction methods. My friends' attitudes were constant, so I retreated from conversations, missed outings, and refrained from attending holiday dinners to avoid criticism.

As mentioned by Corrigan and Associates, "You start to believe through the actions and comments of others."

I had to use crutches for years. People in my apartment house would not help me carry bags, move out of the way, carry trash down the stairs, and excluded me at social functions. The public opened doors for me but kept their eyes down or reached to catch me when I was getting out of a car. Comments included "Be careful," "Live with it," "You will never be the same," etc. These attitudes reinforce your self-belief that you are different.

Fighting back: In 2012, I attempted to play tennis with my young neighbor attending MIT. To my amazement, although my leg was dragging and I could not pivot, I won the match! It became apparent that my backswing had slowed down, which allowed me more control of the tennis ball's placement. Then I attempted to bowl. I fell twice and stopped the game. On my second attempt at bowling, I scored 146. The bowling alley management was so impressed they gave me the ball. Years later, I was promoted to second-degree black belt in karate with limited martial arts.

After the hip infections were gone, I eliminated the use of oxy within a month. I could walk again, even though my spine had deteriorated so much that most activities were limited. I was self-aware of self-stigma by having experienced long-term trauma and pain, which helped me come to grips with this type of stigma. Should you develop self-stigma, attempt to reverse other peoples' attitudes with the self-awareness to laugh at careless comments and focus on activity within your abilities. You will be surprised at what you can achieve, which will improve your self-worth and accomplishments. By observing how you overcome debilitating illness, people who shunned you will begin to come around.

Mark S. fought back by providing positive feedback to home health aides and family. He would work from his house while keeping a cheerful demeanor and optimistic outlook. The stigma that his family induced became irrelevant.

Mentalhealth.org suggests, "The way to fight self-stigma is to identify people who are positive and supportive in your life and spend more time with them. Take less notice of those who run you down. Try to notice and value your strengths."

Mayoclinic.org suggests the following ways to confront self-stigma:

- Get treatment, even if you are reluctant to admit you need treatment.
- Do not let stigma create self-doubt and shame. Stigma does not just come from others.
- Do not isolate yourself.
- Do not equate yourself with your illness.
- Join a support group.
- Speak out against stigma.

Social stigma: Definitions.net defines *social stigma* as "[t]he extreme disapproval of a person or group on socially characteristic grounds that are perceived and serve to distinguish them, from other society members. Stigma may then be affixed to such a person, by the greater society, who differs from their cultural norms."

The perception of others who are healthy, active, and have jobs can overwhelm you as feeling different. That creates "social distancing" — from a trauma or stigma perspective, not the current reference to managing the COVID-19 pandemic. Infection from a medical procedure creates a different environment for you to survive. Pat Sr., Larry, and I are examples of social stigma victims, along with my friend wounded in Kuwait and Peter, who had a stroke. We lost our jobs or livelihoods because of events beyond our control. In a few cases, the lack of self-esteem led to using alcohol or drugs to reduce physical pain and mental stress.

At that point, you do not belong to the culture you were once part of. Your limited or changed world may be defined as "The Subculture," a term defined in Brian Masters' book, *Road to Addiction — Highways to Recovery — The Brian Masters Story*. These individuals fought back even despite having deformities and a life of pain. But the stigma created by others through comments like, "You are an alcoholic," "You are an addict," or "this job requires lifting and walking, so you can't do it" will continue. We cannot hide from it.

However, even with the struggles of social stigma, individuals understand. So many individuals in the medical professional front line have seen so much or have had friends, family, or themselves experience what you have gone through. They have empathy.

A good example is my primary doctor's office. Dr. Ford, Chris, Bani, and the others maintain the health of so many at their UMass, MetroWest office. I became homeless and dependent. **Years later, when I moved past all of that but again was crippled from hip operations, those medical professionals were there for me and never judged me.**

It is not the medical professional's job to care and understand; that cannot be taught. Like Alexa, the RN from the Millbury rehabilitation facility, it comes from within. They are out there. You may be down, but with their help, you are not out.

Fighting back: The TMS Institute of America suggests five ways to fight social stigma.

1. Talk openly about stigma — If you currently suffer from pain due to an illness, share your experiences with others and social media. Talk about how you have learned to cope effectively and what treatment or therapy has worked for you.

2. Understand, educate, and encourage equality between mental and physical health. They are interconnected, and one can significantly influence the other.

3. Show compassion and empathy toward others with stigma due to pain and illness and encourage others to do the same. Today, more than ever before, people do not fight fair. Instead, they bully and post hurtful things about others on social media. People do not understand, care, or think about how these terrible acts affect the well-being of others.

4. Educate yourself about mental health and share your knowledge with others. Understand that even family members and friends may be suffering in silence, which is dangerous.

5. Become your mental health advocate and encourage others to do the same. Take care of your mental health, your illness, and your pain as a result.

Infections

Medicinenet.com defines *infection* as "[t]he invasion and multiplication of micro-organisms such as bacteria, viruses, and parasites that are not normally present within the body. An infection may cause no symptoms and be sub-clinical, or it may cause symptoms and be clinically apparent. An infection may remain localized, or it may spread through the blood or lymphatic vessels to become body-wide."

The infection section complements the decisions that you will have to make. First and foremost, you need to know the risk of being in a hospital and rehabilitation facility. Second, you should know where to look for the information you need, questions to ask at medical consultations, and prevention steps. **Finally, infection prevention is why it is imperative to you, your family, and friends seek multiple opinions.**

Statistics, research, and infection recommendations: The latest CDC statistics reinforce the importance of making educated decisions and obtaining second and third opinions. The information provided below does not reflect the deaths due to COVID-19. Still, they support that you need to investigate the why, where, and who questions to prevent complications from surgery and rehabilitation. Questions, onsite visits, and medical options can save your life. You can find the information you need at https://www.cdc.gov/VitalSigns/staph/.

In 2017, 119,000 patients caught staph infections from medical procedures, and 20,000 patients died from bloodstream staph

infections. My first and second hip infections were due to the left hip implant in 2015 and the right hip implant in 2017. The timing of the operations and statistics were eventful, but there was hope. As I should have done in the first place, acquiring multiple opinions would have given me a fighting chance. In 2018, I, fortunately, interviewed three hospitals and surgeons. I choose two surgeons — Billy Henderson, MD and Dr. Patrick A., and Dr. June Wind, an infectious disease doctor. They saved my life.

The following breakdown for infection risk provides direction questions to ask your surgeons and what your behavior should be.

At UMass Memorial in Worcester, Massachusetts, the orthopedic department has created a database for research, analytics, and reports on surgeons, processes, and patients. The website, Function and Outcomes Research for Comparative Effectiveness in Total Joint Replacement (FORCE-TJR) is the first nationwide comprehensive registry of total joint replacement (TJR) surgical and patient-reported outcomes.

The Force-TJR website states, "Over … five years, under the leadership of Dr. Patricia Franklin and Dr. David Ayers, we collected outcomes from a national mix of surgeons and patients (more than 30,000 patients in total). We developed tools and expertise in PRO data collection, analysis, and reporting in the process. Our methods reflect survey response rates as high as 85% and our analyses offer the unique ability to compare risk-adjusted TJR outcomes to a truly representative national benchmark."

Surgeons' public webcasts are increasing, mainly due to COVID-19 patients who have had surgery and must prepare for home physical therapy days after surgery to avoid the cost and the probability of infections from rehabilitation facilities. If you cannot go home, they suggest going to a relative or an advocate's home until outpatient therapy is completed. Although Force TJR is centered around orthopedics, the organization may provide information that your primary care doctors and surgeons would find helpful outside of UMass. (https://force-tjr.org/about)

Safety for the patient: Doctor Hoffer's book, *Prescription for Bankruptcy, America's Failing Health Care System,* talks about his knowledge of infections. Doctor Hoffer writes, "If you can stay away from a hospital, you should do so. Hospitals are teeming with bad bugs — bacteria highly resistant to antibiotics; these are spread from one patient to another. To recover from an illness or surgery, you need adequate sleep and good nutrition."

We can safely assume that extended stays at rehabilitation facilities fall into Dr. Hoffer's opinions. He does agree that standard infection precautions such as these will help.

Centers for Disease Control: Morbidity and Mortality Weekly Report (MMWR), March 2019 — "What puts people at risk for a serious staph infection?"

In communities:

- Uncovered or draining wounds, especially in high-contact sports or crowded living conditions

- Sharing personal items, such as towels or razors
- Recent stays in a healthcare facility
- Injection drug use, such a heroin

In hospitals:

- Hospital stays or surgery (during and shortly after)
- Sharing personal items, such as towels or razors
- Exposure to patients carrying or infected with staph
- Medical devices in the body, such as intravenous lines (IVs) and implants

In other healthcare facilities:

- Outpatient surgery and procedures, such as dialysis
- Nursing homestays
- Medical devices in the body, such s IVs

Due diligence in educating yourself about infections and prevention is the best way to reduce the probability of contracting germs that lead to infection and pain. The Joint Commission website and Medicare.gov/compare will help you know if a hospital has the best credentials for your situation. Your primary doctor and surgeon should also have access to more detailed information through the Joint Commission website. Target a hospital's infection rate and ask the medical professionals to access www.qualitycheck.org and www.thejointcommission.org.

There is a friend — the Infectious Disease Doctor: webmd.com defines the infectious disease doctor as "a physician who specializes in the various infections that can

> affect the human body. An infectious disease doctor may also be known as an ID physician. There is a great deal of overlap with microbiologists who specialize in infections as well, although ID physicians tend to focus more clinically."

The infectious disease doctor is one of the specialties you never hear about until you need them. When you become ill and the specialty doctor orders that you visit the infectious disease doctor, the first-time visitor will ask, "Who is that and what do they do?" Well, they save your life or reduce your pain and misery — if possible.

I can only speak from my experience. I had two such doctors: Dr. Lopez at UMass and Dr. Wind from Newton Wellesley. In 2017, when the pain from the first hip infection became unbearable, Dr. Lopez knew what to prescribe and how it would work with the infection. As a result, I was able to function normally until the second hip infection. Then, Dr. Wind saved my life after surgeons in other hospitals had made their mistakes. Dr. Wind was the doctor who ordered the last four applications of the antibiotic Vancomycin before I was discharged from the rehab facility and traveled to Newton for aspirations on both hips to see if the infections were eliminated. Thus, both infectious disease doctors saved me from a world of pain and death.

If you must investigate the infectious disease doctor's expertise from the tools mentioned in the book, do it thoroughly.

Interestingly, both doctors continued to follow up and see how I was doing a year after being released from their responsibility. I would often answer the phone and hear Dr. Lopez's voice, asking how things were going. Same with Dr. Wind. That cannot be taught. It is a function of the doctor's character and genuine interest in your wellbeing. It reminded me of the 1970's TV show Dr. Marcus Welby, M.D., starring Robert Young, James Brolin, and Elena Verdugo; personal follow-up rarely happens these days.

Patient's infection experiences: The risk of infection can be reduced by using current prevention procedures before and after surgery. An example would be bathing with the prescribed medical soap, liberally, five days before your surgery. However, the fact remains that statistics show that infection is probable because of hospital and rehabilitation processes and environments.

Consider orthopedic procedures in 2019. There were 600,000 implants, of whom 375,000 had hip replacements. Any information can be relevant to this large population. In a 2017 study by *MicrobiologyOpen*, 56.1% of implants showed staphylococci from these operations.

I contracted *Staphylococcus bacteremia* during the 2011 surgery spine operation, complicated by nosocomial pneumonia and acute pleural necrosis. *Bacteremia,* according to freedictionary.com/bacterium, is "a common infectious cause of morbidity and mortality worldwide, causing both community-acquired and hospital-acquired bacteremia. In the U.S. alone, it accounts for 23% of all bloodstream infections and is the bacterial pathogen most strongly associated with death."

In 2015 and 2017, I had no choice but to have my hips replaced. Unfortunately, I contracted *Coagulase*—negative staph in the right hip in the 2017 operation and *Enterobacter cloaca* in the left hip during the 2015 operation.

According to *Microbewiki,* the 2015 operation was responsible for infections such as bacteremia, lower respiratory tract infections, skin and soft tissue infections, urinary tract infections, endocarditis, intra-abdominal infections, septic arthritis, osteomyelitis, and ophthalmic infections.

The 2017 operation infection, according to *Microbewiki,* was the effect of "nosocomial pathogens that can cause a range of infections such as bacteremia, lower respiratory tract infection, skin and soft tissue infections, urinary tract infections, endocarditis, intra-abdominal infections, septic arthritis, osteomyelitis, and ophthalmic infections," commonly acquired during hospitalization."

They were* bacteremia *infections contracted in a hospital environment, and they are deadly. I was fortunate to live through the infections with the help of my chosen surgeons, infectious disease doctor, and advocates.

While at a casino, a man named Steve asked me why I walked "weird." We talked, and I told him my story. Steve said, "I thought that might have been the problem: hospitals and infection." Steve told me about his sister, who had a standard operation on her stomach at a hospital in Lowell, Massachusetts, but contracted a fast-moving infection and died within two weeks.

Occasionally, even the best hospitals listed in *Medicare.gov/comparehospitals* and the Joint Commission fail the patient. For example, my friend Pat Sr. from the YMCA lost a leg from infections that started from his ankle implant and spread to the knee at a highly accredited hospital in Boston that treats Boston's top athletes. He had no choice but to have his leg removed below the knee. Pat Sr. had been a master in the martial arts style of Chin Ru and held the rank of fourth-degree black belt, but he lost his livelihood due to infection. He survived, drives, and lives a good life but is in constant pain.

Pat Sr. continues to battle pain, especially when he attempts to sleep. He learned that I also suffer daily, so he suggested Veterinary Liniment Gel for the pain area. It worked better than drugs and Tylenol for arthritis. Thank Pat Sr. if it works for you.

The significant amount of time I spent in hospitals and rehabilitation care has provided me this opportunity to write about men and women who suffered from infections because of hospital or rehabilitation facility stays. They know other people who have been infected. The total number of stories becomes exponential.

Methods of infection prevention: The cdc.gov website is a wealth of knowledge about infection prevention. Its research can help you focus on infection prevention for your diagnosed illness. My infection was contracted in the operating room. The CDC article about hospital environmental causes and infection prevention supports the unfortunate outcome. Understanding why infections occur and why hospitals do not invest in preventing them can influence the critical decision you have to make. The CDC writes:

> **Through population movement, infections from the operating room:** "Operating room air may contain micro-organisms, dust, aerosol, lint, skin squamous epithelial cells, and respiratory droplets. The microbial level in operating room air is directly proportional to the number of people moving in the room. One study documented lower infection rates with coagulase-negative staphylococci among patients when operating room traffic during the surgical procedure was limited. Therefore, efforts should be made to minimize personnel traffic during operations. Outbreaks of SSIs caused by group A beta-hemolytic streptococci have been traced to airborne transmission from colonized operating-room personnel to patients. Several potential healthcare-associated pathogens (e.g., *Staphylococcus aureus* and *Staphylococcus epidermidis*) and drug-resistant organisms have also been recovered in areas adjacent to the surgical field, but the extent to which the presence of bacteria near the surgical field influences the development of post-operative SSIs is not clear.
>
> "Proper ventilation, humidity (< 68%), and temperature control in the operating room are important for the comfort

of surgical personnel and patients, but also in preventing environmental conditions that encourage growth and transmission of micro-organisms."
(https://www.cdc.gov/infectioncontrol/guidelines/environmental/background/air.html#c5c)

Yet, the hospital system and medical reimbursements financially hamstring infection safety. In "The Incremental Cost of infections Associated with Multidrug-Resistant Organisms in the Inpatient Hospital Setting-A National Estimate," Kenton Johnson and partners discuss the financial reasoning behind why medical facilities do not invest more money and effort to reduce Hospital Acquired Infections (HAIs). "This study is to simulate incentives for reducing hospital-acquired infections under various payment configurations by Medicare, Medicaid, and private payers." Their conclusion was, "Higher markups help hospitals earn positive margins and retain earnings for capital investments needed to reduce infection. Broadly increasing payment rates reduces the incentives for hospitals to invest in quality improvement measures that lead to a reduction in healthcare costs."

Medical payments and reimbursements are the keys to preventing HAIs, which leaves us helpless when preventing hospital infection decisions.

A 2018 research paper in *Infection Control & Hospital Epidemiology*, "Financial Incentives to Reduce Hospital-Acquired Infections Under Alternative Payment Arrangements," concludes, "hospital incentives for investing in patient safety vary by payer and payment configuration. Higher payments provide resources to improve patient safety, but the current payment structures may also reduce the willingness of hospitals to invest in patient safety."

I have researched and read medical reports for years. One reason was to understand what was done to me and who fixed it. The other was to pass on what I learned through this book. So when I drilled down into studies about infections and how they are given to us, I decided to write what I think may have happened in 2011.

The surgeon, the nurses, an anesthesiologist, instrument support, and potentially a second surgeon are in the operating room. In my case, I had my spine operation at a well-known teaching hospital. When I would take my son to the facility in the past for outpatient procedures, the doctors would ask if the residents could be present and learn. Of course, we would say *yes* and think nothing of it. Now, patients and medical professionals are confident that an increase in the number of individuals in the operating room increases the chance of infection from air currents, people's movements, and limited ventilation.

The hospital operation reports that Don Hanssen and I read years later only provided the doctor's name who wrote the report, not the number of medical professionals present at the time. It is an important question that you/we should ask before each operation. **How many and who are they? After**

each operation, you/we should ask how many medical professionals were present and who were they? Your life could depend on it.

Understanding the Diagnosis-Related Group (DRG): How does the patient prevent the internal health systems incentive costs and issues affecting their surgeries, and ultimately their quality of life? It could be as simple as understanding the DRG system in the healthcare process and the specialist's coding for maximum insurance coverage.

HMSA.com says the DRG system can help the patient "speak intelligently to surgeons, specialists, and the staff that bill the health care provider."

"A diagnosis-related group (DRG) is a patient classification system that standardizes prospective payment to hospitals and encourages cost containment initiatives. In general, a DRG payment covers all charges associated with an inpatient stay from the time of admission to discharge. The DRG payment system is reflected in the increased efficiency and transparency of patient care".

"An advantage of DRG is a reduced average length of stay, which reduces the risk of infections. The disadvantage of DRG is creating financial incentives toward earlier hospital discharges. Occasionally, such policies are not in full accordance with the clinical benefit priorities." (May 12, 2016)

DRGs have historically been used for inpatient care. Still, the 21st Century Cures Act, enacted in late 2016, required the

Centers for Medicare and Medicaid Services to develop some DRGs that also apply to outpatient surgeries.

Combining the selection of surgeons, hospitals, rehabilitation facilities (if needed), and knowledge of DRG and its effect on maximum coverage and care should reduce the incidence of hospital infections. Ideally, by working with the specialist and their staff for appropriate short- or long-term care, you can be assured in full accordance with clinical benefit priorities.

After reading this book, you should now investigate the websites I have mentioned. You should refer to the websites of the hospital and rehabilitation facilities you are choosing for verification of accreditation by the Joint Commission and combine your investigation by using the Medicare.gov/compare database, which provides valuable reports.

The Newton hospital and its medical professionals that helped me overcome the infections that I contracted at a South Coast hospital freely post their recognition of infection prevention by the Joint Commission on their website.

Summary of 2019 Joint Commission Findings

The Joint Commission (TJC) conducted its three-year reaccreditation survey of Newton-Wellesley Hospital (NWH) from November 12–15, 2019. A team of five TJC surveyors — consisting of two registered nurses, two physicians, and one life safety engineer — visited NWH's main campus and offsite locations for the unannounced, four-day survey. The surveyors' objectives were to:

- Validate NWH's compliance with standards and provide a meaningful assessment of risks.
- Inspire and encourage improvement through engagement and dialogue.
- Partner on the journey toward becoming a high-reliability organization.

During their evaluation, the survey team identified areas of improvement that they have been working to address, including:

- Infection control — standardizing processes and consistently adhering to hospital policies and manufacturers' recommendations.
- Suicide prevention — ensuring the highest level of safety for patients at risk for suicide.
- Physical environment — optimizing procedures and processes for maintenance to support the safest physical environment for patients, visitors, and staff.

TJC conducted a follow-up survey on December 27, 2019, to evaluate initial improvements, which is standard practice and typical for most hospitals. The follow-up visit was a success and concluded the onsite survey component of the institution's triennial accreditation.

Cross-checking your chosen hospital's websites should confirm your investigation. The positive outcome at the hospital's website is impressive but is only their opinion. Cross-check with medicare.gov/compare, sites mentioned in the book, and resources provided by the medical community.

Your family and friends may be limited by resource availability, which may hinder your options search. The first hospital where I had my hip operations provided no such information at that time or currently. As I suggest in the decision-making sessions for your investigation techniques, use the question checklist.

I must reiterate that my book provides valuable, real-life information for your path through the surgical procedures, hospitals, rehabilitation, and home care processes.

Every town, city, and country has varied resources, so they may not pertain to every reader. Hospital and rehabilitation facilities may be limited in your area. Insurance and medical healthcare coverage differ from person to person but investing time and money to investigate hospital, and surgical options must be a priority for you, even if you must travel or pay more to expand insurance coverage. Chapters of this book will pertain to anyone having to rely on the medical world and those who make medical decisions.

By considering more than one doctor, hospital, or rehabilitation facility, you will save yourself a life of agony. Many in this book, including myself, chose not to investigate different opinions and suffered infections, pain, unnecessary operations, social stigma, and disability for life. Following the information in this book "*Navigate the Medical Maze*" will lead you to think of options and in-depth investigation before making medical procedure decisions. Should you have learned anything from all or parts of the book, it has accomplished its intention.

We must remember to Hope — Fight — Live.

WILLIAM REILEY BUTLER

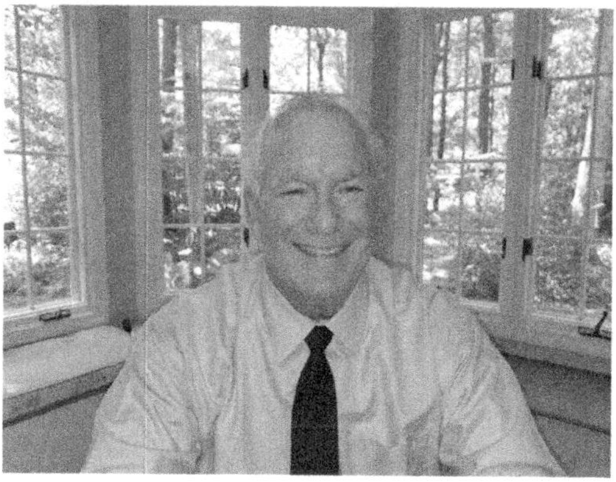

William Reiley Butler, was raised in Fayetteville-Manlius, New York and now resides in Massachusetts.

He was an honor student at Syracuse University, a successful high technology sales executive, has a son, Billy in Hollywood, and holds a 2nd degree Black Belt in Ed Parkers Kenpo Karate.

Years later, after multiple operations, he contracted infections in the spine, hips, and legs from botched medical procedures, resulting in consistent chronic pain.

William is the author of nonfiction books that focus on real life stories, informed information, and help towards critical life decisions. His first book created eleven action plans for the homeless and those affected by substance abuse. The book has been endorsed by top experts in the field.

This second book is meant to provide direction in advocacy, choices in healing, understanding pain communication, and taking control of your decisions.

He is a patron of FreeLancewiting, NY Book Editors, Authors Learning Center, Patient and Healthcare Advocacy, and Saint Vincent DePaul. The Life's Realities website is william-butler.com. His blog complementing the first book, www.addictionrealityeducation.com, exposes the realities of substance abuse and promotes uplifting results through education and multiple recovery solutions.

PLEASE RATE MY BOOK

I would be very grateful if you would please take a few moments to rate my book on Amazon.com (U.S.).

Or, if you're in any of these countries, please use these Amazon sites:

Amazon.ca (Canada)
Amazon.com.au (Australia)
Amazon.de (Germany)
Amazon.com.mx (Mexico)
Amazon.co.uk (U.K.)
Amazon.fr (France)
Amazon.co.jp (Japan)
Amazon.es (Spain)

A 5-star rating *and* a short review (e.g. "Jam-packed with valuable strategies!" or "Many people I know need this book!") would be much appreciated. We welcome longer, positive comments as well.

If you feel like this book should be rated at three stars or fewer, please hold off posting your comments on Amazon. Instead, please send your feedback directly to me, so that we can use it to improve the next edition. We're committed to providing the best value to our customers and readers, and your thoughts can make that possible.

You can reach me at william-butler.com.

Thank you.
Keep smiling!,

William Reiley Butler

Publisher-Author
Life's Realities Press

Made in the USA
Monee, IL
04 November 2026

67385943R10115